With a Light Touch is full of gracious ╲
geriatric medicine who has fully integrated
and skill with the faith that energises him. Iι
and compassion and has given us a deeply encouraging book full of
practical help, backed by fascinating research and years of experience. I
came away informed, cheered and renewed in hope.

Bishop John Pritchard

The title of Ian's book perfectly expresses the way in which he has
given us a most thoughtful and perceptive introduction to a subject which
must concern us all.

He does this from his long experience as a physician specialising in
'frailty'. This term in itself reminds us that vulnerability and dependence
are not the preserve of the elderly. Individual independence is an illusion.

Ian's deep Christian faith undergirds this book, but it is never partisan
or hectoring. He has a large view of healing, reminding us that it is not
all about 'curing'. Bringing wholeness can mean 'making sense and
coming to terms with our condition, improving the symptoms so that we
can live with it; and even using it for a new purpose'. His approach to
dying and death is similarly creative.

This is indeed a book for our time and I am sure it will both encourage
and challenge all who read it.

Canon Neil Heavisides

This book wonderfully fills a gap on many bookshelves. It is born
from years of experience and a deep Christian faith. The pages of this
book dare to name things that are often not spoken, and Ian Donald
weaves together the practical and the reflective. Whether you are
someone in the later years of life, a family member or carer, or someone
who is having the courage to think about what it means to grow old, this
book is a treasure trove of wisdom, pertinent questions and pragmatic
comment, all rooted in the bigger picture of what it means to be mortal.

The Rt Revd Rachel Treweek
Bishop of Gloucester and Anglican Bishop for HM Prisons

Dr Ian Donald is a geriatrician who brings many years of experience in working with frailty to this book. It's a superb book. I only wish we'd had something like it when my dad lived with us. I think it will benefit both carers and those of us who are 'getting on a bit'! It needs to be read by anyone who looks after elderly relatives, or as a preparation for our own aging and dying.

The blend of Christian teaching and thinking and the medical perspective is so helpful – and excellent.

I highly recommend it.

Sheila Appleton

RGN (Retired), Adv. Dip. Pastoral Counselling (Nottingham University), Post qualifying cert (Adlerian), BACP Registered Accredited Counsellor

The book covers an important subject in a compassionate and clear way. It is wide-ranging in terms of considering the issues affecting the fourth age, and the use of 'real-life' examples add validity to the subject matter as one knows that they are based on a genuine professional experience. As a clinician I have long thought that some of the care we provide for the older population is over-medicalised and has also not always been completely person-centred. This book cogently explains how more holistic approaches are far more appropriate, and that when they are underpinned by a Jesus-centred attitude and philosophy, it is possible to age well and, indeed, die well in our post-modern society.

Dr Andrew Seymour

GP and Chair of Gloucestershire Clinical Commissioning Group

Ian has been an advocate for older people for many years; his passion has been plain to see. This book is a distillation of his knowledge and his faith, written in a style that makes the information accessible to all...

Prof. David G Smithard MD FRCP FRCSLT (Hon)

Editor, Triple Helix, Christian Medical Fellowship

About the Author

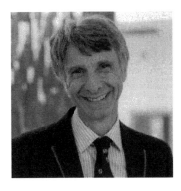

Dr Ian Donald trained at Cambridge and Edinburgh Universities, and became a consultant in Geriatric Medicine in Gloucester in 1988. He led the department for fifteen years and undertook research into the epidemiology of ageing within the county, which led to over twenty publications and his MD at Cambridge University. Throughout his career he was a pioneer for hospital-at-home services and liaison healthcare with care homes and community teams, and in the last ten years he developed a specialist frailty team working in the emergency department of the hospital.

He became concerned that many older people were taking too many medications potentially causing more harm than good, and this led to the development of his own prescribing guidelines for those living with frailty. These were widely adopted across the county and led to marked improvements in appropriate prescribing. In 2018 the Gloucestershire Hospitals Trust chose him for the Lifetime Achievement Award. He has been a member of the Christian Medical Fellowship throughout his working career, and was invited to speak at the New Wine conferences in 2009 and 2010 on some of the topics raised in his book, *With a Light Touch*.

His wife of forty years, Philippa, was ordained in the Church of England in 2011. They have three sons and two grand-daughters.

To contact the author, please write to: *ecare@blueyonder.co.uk*

More information about the author can be found on the book's web page:

www.onwardsandupwards.org/with-a-light-touch

With A Light Touch

A guide to healthcare in frailty

Dr Ian Donald

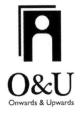

O&U
Onwards & Upwards

Onwards and Upwards Publishers

4 The Old Smithy, London Road, Rockbeare,
EX5 2EA, United Kingdom.
www.onwardsandupwards.org

First edition, published in the United Kingdom by Onwards and Upwards Publishers (2021).

ISBN: 978-1-78815-929-6
Illustrator: Benjamin Harris
Typeface: Sabon LT

This book is dedicated to:

the wonderful and inspiring frailty team
at Gloucestershire Royal Hospital
and the county's community matrons

and my wife Philippa
for her belief in this project.

Contents

With A Light Touch

Introduction

The LORD is my light and salvation: whom shall I fear?[1]

HER FUNERAL WAS MEMORABLE, BUT NOT BECAUSE SHE WAS a celebrity or locally famous. There was no horse-drawn hearse or procession through the streets; there were no outlandish costumes or exceptional displays of flowers. I was playing the organ for the Anglican service – as a consultant in geriatric medicine, many local funerals will be for patients I have known and treated, but I was here as a close friend of the family rather than because of a professional connection. I had attended to her professionally twice – the first time was to conduct a thorough medication review, adjusting her pills to the ones that would maximise wellbeing, and discarding many others; the second time was nearer the end of her life when we all thought she might be dying. It was around Christmas, and she was very unwell with a pneumonia, but she did not wish to go into hospital. I changed her antibiotics, and by some good fortune, but more likely the hand of God, she rallied. I visited her on Christmas Eve to find her sitting up in bed, organising the family, and she did not die until the following Easter. Let me tell you something about her.

Joy was a supreme example of someone who lived life to the full. Diminutive in size and bent over due to a crumbling of the spine, she remained cheerful, energetic and positive into old age, rising early and going to bed late. Sharp as a tack, with a prodigious memory, she was determined to pack each precious day of her life as full as possible, seeing as many people as possible, which she continued to do until her death at the age of ninety-two.

Joy's attitude was that life was for *living!* Her deep Christian faith was the bedrock of her life and it sustained her every day. Her personal journey of faith began as a teenager, and from then on she always had what she called her 'quiet time' first thing every morning, reading the Bible and praying.

Joy's home was always full of people of all ages, ethnicities and cultures, and everyone was welcomed with open arms and loving

---

[1] Psalm 27:1 (NIV)

hospitality. ("Oh, you must have another piece of flapjack!") She would draw them out, listening and affirming as they talked, then praying for them later. Her home was packed with furniture, photos of her extensive family, mementos of her life. There were some physical hazards there – a geriatrician's nightmare! – but her interest in and love of people always came first. In spite of frailty, she travelled widely until the end of her life to visit friends she had made and cherished, and would not be put off. If a wheelchair was needed, for speed and ease, so be it. The Christmas before she died, she was very ill and could not leave her bedroom, so the family brought Christmas to her there. After Christmas, she was heard to comment, "Well, God must have some more praying for me to do, then!" which she did until she died the following Easter. On the morning of the day, she read her Bible verse for the day which said, "Enter now into the joy of the Lord" – and she did. Joy was an inspiration to everyone who knew her.

Is this something that we aspire to? A life remaining productive in God's eyes in spite of disability, with strong binds of love across the generations? This book is about the time in your life when you are no longer independent but rely on help from others. We love to celebrate a long life, but most of us try to avoid the thought of dependency, because it is too fearful – fear of pain, or indignity, or loss of identity and value, and becoming a burden on others. In fact, dependence on each other is what makes us human – we were created for relationship. Think of Adam and Eve. Humans are born very dependent, become independent, and may re-enter a second period of dependency.

This book will refer frequently to the notion of 'frailty' – a time defined by vulnerability and dependency. Geriatrics is my medical specialty, which has grown rapidly through the second half of the twentieth century in recognition of the special medical needs of those living with frailty. It is centred on the belief that old people are valuable. It believes that healthcare can ease the experience of ageing but knows that too much medicine can worsen that experience.

Older people have grown up with respect for doctors – a 'doctor knows best' attitude – and take the prescribed pills often having no idea what they are for! It can seem to them disrespectful to refuse the doctor's advice. We may be swept along by the medical train – what starts as a phone call to the GP or NHS Direct, turns into a blood test, a hospital attendance, and then an admission, and then scans, and then being told what needs to be done or what pills we need to take. The whole process is driven by evidence-based guidelines developed for younger people. Yet for those living with frailty, those guidelines don't quite work – they were not designed with frailty in mind – and could even do more harm than good. So, we may need to break the rules a bit and use a lighter, gentler approach.

Modern healthcare is quite remarkable and has so much to offer us over the later years of life. Annual health expenditure on an eighty-year-old in the UK is more than five times the expenditure on a fifty-year-old. In the last year of life, the health costs for that eighty-year-old are fourfold higher again. Is some of this expenditure trying to halt a tide that cannot be stemmed? Christians can be drawn into placing their hope and trust in healthcare rather than in Jesus Christ for the future. It takes courage to face up to the realities of ageing – "Old age ain't no place for sissies!" (Bette Davis); it takes courage to be honest about the risks and limitations of healthcare, and it takes courage to let go. There are enough challenges to living with frailty. Healthcare should be there to help with those challenges without being a burden at the same time. There is a widespread concern that healthcare may be unwisely used to prolong the dying process. Atul Gawande, an American surgeon, wrote in his celebrated book *Being Mortal:*

> *...people live longer and better than at any other time in history. But scientific advances have turned the process of ageing and dying into medical experiences, matters to be managed by health care professionals. ... This experiment of making mortality a medical experience is just decades old. It is young. And the evidence is it is failing.*[2]

There is no doubt that medicine today has the ability to prolong life, but sometimes that extra life may not seem worth living. Over my working lifetime, there have been times when a patient has asked me if I could end things for them, and those requests have seemed to come more frequently in recent years. An online survey in 2019 of over five thousand people believed to be representative of the UK population showed eighty-four percent supported legalised euthanasia. I believe the principal reasons driving this support are the fear that medicine might keep us alive well beyond the time we would wish, and the fear of lost personhood

---

[2]   Atul Gawande (2014); *Being Mortal;* Profile Books

through dementia. A traumatic family experience witnessing a spiral of decline will probably shape our views about euthanasia. Does it have to be like this? Are we making mortality a medical experience? Could we end our lives more naturally?

I have been convinced that with more honest and courageous joint decision-making a little earlier on, doctors and patients can recognise together when healthcare has become an intrusive burden. Such an understanding can reduce the chance of a prolonged final illness in hospital, and thus quieten the cry for legalising euthanasia. I found that those difficult but frank conversations are generally welcomed. We will explore this in the later chapters of the book. This is part of the 'letting go', when we honestly face up to the facts and accept that further treatment will not help.

Over the following chapters, I will lift the lid on aspects of healthcare for older people, which I hope will help you use healthcare more wisely. I will explain what doctors mean by 'frailty' because it is principally to those supporting someone with frailty that I write. We are instructed to honour our father and mother; older people are often proud, resisting help, combined with a stubbornness perhaps acquired from living through the war. I will suggest when becoming involved in their medical care is the right thing to do, even if it leads to an argument. I will explain the value of a careful review of all the medications taken; 'deprescribing' with fewer pills can actually improve health! Blood tests and scans are often essential to understanding symptoms, but I will explore the pitfalls of overdiagnosis and chasing certainty. There can seem little choice going into hospital in an emergency, but I will explore where there may be alternatives and the reasons why getting back home as soon as possible is usually the best thing. There are pointers to asking the right questions at every encounter. In the later chapters I will explore how to make decisions ahead of time that have a realistic chance of influencing the sort of care received approaching the end of life. Living with dementia is another thread running throughout the book and poses particular challenges in healthcare decision-making and respecting personhood.

The apostle Paul was able to acknowledge frailty coexisting with the imminent journey into eternity:

> *Therefore we do not lose heart. Though outwardly we are wasting away, yet inwardly we are being renewed day by day. For our light and momentary troubles are achieving for*

us an eternal glory that far outweighs them all. So we fix our eyes not on what is seen, but on what is unseen, since what is seen is temporary, but what is unseen is eternal.[3]

We can try more pills, undergo more tests and spend longer in hospital in the hope that all will be well again. But for those living with frailty there are diminishing returns. There comes a time when, with humility, we must admit that too much medicine is doing more harm than good and a lighter touch is required. So now let's explore how healthcare can best be used through the years of frailty.

---

[3] 2 Corinthians 4:16-18 (NIV)

With A Light Touch

CHAPTER ONE

The Realities of Ageing – How Did We Get Here?

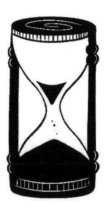

So teach us to number our days aright, that we may gain a heart of wisdom.[4]

WHEN BEING INTRODUCED AT SOCIAL GATHERINGS, ONE OF the most common questions I am asked as a geriatrician is, "So when do I get counted as geriatric?" The questioner is of course hoping for an answer that is at least ten years above their current age. Then perhaps they can relax and put off for a bit longer any thoughts that one day they might be anything less than fully independent. By contrast, the geriatrician in me is looking around the house and wondering how adaptable this house might be if a stroke or broken hip should come along.

None of us likes to think we are getting older. Of course, we still feel the same inside – but we can see that our friends look older! We live in an ageing society, by which we mean that the proportion of the

---

[4]   Psalm 90:12 (NIV)

population who are over sixty-five keeps increasing. You and I, as individuals, are able to enjoy the benefits of this ageing society: with improved life expectancy, most of us can look forward to enjoying many years after retirement in comparatively good health and wealth. Many of today's retired population have benefited from final salary pension schemes and the 'triple lock' state pension in the UK which have exceeded inflation for many years, although such generosity may not continue much longer and around a fifth of the over eighty-fives today live in poverty.[5]

The process and experience of ageing was not unfamiliar to the people of the Old Testament in the Bible; the description of the physical impact of ageing found in Ecclesiastes certainly pulls no punches. The text vividly describes the later years of life and the perils of frailty, revealing that old age was understood three thousand years ago:

When you get old,
  the light from the sun, moon, and stars will grow dark;
  the rain clouds will never seem to go away.
At that time your arms will shake
  and your legs will become weak.
Your teeth will fall out so you cannot chew,
  and your eyes will not see clearly.
Your ears will be deaf to the noise in the streets,
  and you will barely hear the millstone grinding grain.
You'll wake up when a bird starts singing,
  but you will barely hear singing.
You will fear high places
  and will be afraid to go for a walk.
Your hair will become white like the flowers on an almond tree.
  You will limp along like a grasshopper when you walk.
  Your appetite will be gone.
Then you will go to your everlasting home,
  and people will go to your funeral.[6]

---

[5] Age UK (2020); 'Poverty in Later Life'; ageuk.org.uk; poverty_in_later_life_briefing_june_2019.pdf

[6] Ecclesiastes 12:1-5 (NCV)

It is hardly surprising that such a depressing view of the ageing process will make us try to pretend it will never happen. We comfort ourselves with phrases such as "sixty is the new forty" and "you're only as old as you feel". Interestingly, you probably are as old as you *look* – at least without facial cosmetic surgery; a large Danish twins study showed that observers could predict which twin would live the longest just from photographs of their faces.[7]

Is old age just a state of mind? We may like to think that if we eat well and exercise regularly, perhaps we will be able to fend off old age and disability. The transformation of ageing in the UK through the twentieth century was quite remarkable – the proportion of the population over sixty-five years rose from five to eighteen percent. Life expectancy, which can be defined as the average age at death, steadily increased at the rate of an additional two to three years every decade – in 1901 the average life expectancy at birth was only forty-eight years for men and fifty-two years for women. Now it has reached eighty years for men and eighty-three years for women.[8] And it is still increasing. The most common age at death in 2018 was eighty-six years for men and eighty-eight years for women. The rising life expectancy has slowed a little since 2000 but is still an extra one to two years every decade.

Much of this improved life expectancy relates to the dramatic drop in infant and childhood deaths. Healthcare contributed to this, but improved public health and general living conditions were probably more important. Back in 1900 there were few people who reached the age of sixty-five – those who survived the poor standards of public health – but on reaching sixty-five they could expect to live another twelve years. Now those reaching sixty-five can expect to live on average another twenty-one years.[9]

It is only the population over sixty-five who will see substantial numerical growth in the next twenty years – a rise of thirty-six percent

---

[7] Christensen K *et al* (2009); 'Perceived age as clinically useful biomarker of ageing: a cohort study'; BMJ 2009;339:b5262

[8] Jagger C (2015); 'Trends in life expectancy and healthy life expectancy'; Foresight, government office for science

[9] ONS (2020)
https://www.ons.gov.uk/peoplepopulationandcommunity/birthsdeathsandm arriages/lifeexpectancies/bulletins/pastandprojecteddatafromtheperiodandco hortlifetables/1981to2068#how-has-life-expectancy-changed-for-those-aged-65

of those sixty-five to seventy-nine, and a rise of seventy-two percent of those aged over eighty. There are now already three million people in the UK over eighty years – likely to be five million by 2040. The number of centenarians has risen from around a hundred in 1901 to 13,300 in 2019. The Queen's telegram service is kept very busy – an average of twenty-one every day! Current estimates are that twenty percent of boys born today and twenty-six percent of girls will live to a hundred years.[10]

Is there perhaps a ceiling – a maximum age for humans? The book of Genesis describes some people living hundreds of years. I will not attempt to interpret the apparent huge longevity of some characters in the Genesis story, but many people believe the numbers are symbolic and relate to Babylonian mathematics known as base sixty. Yet it is intriguing that Genesis might suggest a maximum lifespan of 120 years: "My spirit will not contend with man for ever, for he is mortal; his days will be one hundred and twenty years."[11] Outside of Genesis only one Old Testament character is documented to have lived beyond a hundred years – namely Moses who died at 120, apparently escaping the impact of ageing: "when he died, his eyes were not weak nor his strength gone"[12]! The age of the oldest person alive in modern times has increased very slowly through the twentieth century, but there does appear to be a ceiling effect around 120; only one person has been documented to have lived beyond 120 – Jeanne Calment, who died in France aged 122 in 1997. No-one else as far as we know has broken the 120 barrier in the last twenty-three years.

Are these extra years in good health?

Sometimes referred to as the Third Age, the years of retirement now offer multiple opportunities for fulfilment. Of course, what matters most to us is being in 'good enough' health to enjoy those retirement years and do the things we want to: to socialise with friends, to be active, to work in a paid or voluntary capacity, for as long as we want, and to be independent. This is calculated as 'disability-free life expectancy' (DFLE), and this has also been increasing over the last century. At the age of sixty-five in the UK today, DFLE has reached 10.5 years for men and eleven years for women. So, on average we can expect ten healthy years from

10 Ibid.
11 Genesis 6:3 (NIV)
12 Deuteronomy 34:7 (NIV)

sixty-five, assuming good health at the start.[13] Postponing the average age when any disability starts also means that the average eighty-year-old today is fitter than ten or twenty years ago, so that is good news too.[14] The psalmist predicted that if we remain fit, we may hope to live a little longer: "The days of our life are seventy years, or perhaps eighty if we are strong."[15]

And then what? The hope is that not only can we push back the age when we start to experience some disability, but also that we would see a reduction in the number of years when we are not quite so independent. Can healthcare steadily reduce the years spent in poor health before a final decline? This is known as the 'compression of morbidity' theory – an idea proposed by Dr Fries, an American gerontologist.[16] His idea was that if we are much older when we first meet disability, then we might expect to have fewer years of life left to be lived with disability. We are cheered to hear the stories of lives lived to the full – still working their allotment at ninety-two, or running a marathon at one hundred, and then just dying peacefully in their sleep. Unfortunately, although true for some individuals, this compression of morbidity does not seem to be the experience for most, and on average the number of years lived with some limitations is increasing. Sadly, the years free of any disability are not increasing as fast as the years with some limitation, and so the proportion of our retirement spent in full health is actually falling.[17]

Are we living longer because of improved healthcare?

One key question we need to ask in our understanding of healthcare and old age is to what extent modern healthcare is the reason for our ageing society. Is it because of the success of medical care earlier in life

---

[13] Age UK (2019); 'Briefing: Health and care of older people in England'; www.ageuk.org.uk/globalassets/age-uk/documents/ reports-and-publications/reports-and-briefings/health--wellbeing /age_uk_briefing_state_of_health_ and_care_of_older_people_july2019.pdf

[14] Donald IP (2010); 'Trends in disability prevalence over 10 years in older people living in Gloucestershire'; Age Ageing 39:337-342

[15] Psalm 90:10 (NRSV)

[16] Fries, J (1980); 'Ageing, natural death, and the compression of morbidity'; NEJM 303:130-5

[17] Jagger C (2015); 'Trends in life expectancy and healthy life expectancy'; Foresight, government office for science

that more people live for longer than they might wish, with huge dependence on others or in nursing homes?

The extra years in good health from sixty-five are a tribute to good healthcare, but also to improved diet, an active lifestyle and reduction in smoking – public health measures we are all encouraged to follow. In 1950 eighty percent of older men smoked and now only fifteen percent smoke, which has had a profound effect on lung disease such as chronic bronchitis and circulatory diseases. Heart disease increased rapidly after the second world war, but since 1960 there has been a steady but quite dramatic fall. Mortality rates from heart attacks and stroke have each decreased by seventy percent over the last thirty years.[18] Studies across the developed world have found that about half of that improvement in heart disease is due to medical care following angina or a heart attack – for example coronary vessel surgery and stents.[19] The other half is due to better management of cholesterol, blood pressure and reduced smoking. Similarly, for cancer, survival for five years after a diagnosis of cancer in the UK has improved from twenty-five to fifty percent in the last forty years, and this is almost certainly due to improved medical treatment.[20]

So, healthcare has had a major impact in more recent years in reducing premature deaths from diseases such as heart disease and cancer. But is healthcare also contributing to the prolonged years in poor health towards the end of life – potentially keeping people alive beyond their desire? For instance, the successful prevention of deaths from heart attacks has led to a rise in the number of people now living with disability from heart failure – symptoms of a weakened heart after a heart attack. Powerful antibiotics, sometimes by injection, are another healthcare weapon which has had a major impact on those living with frailty. Hospital treatment for pneumonia will often be successful in saving lives, although the benefit may be short-lived. Those with more advanced frailty are susceptible to recurring infections. Indeed, the readmission rate after going home for those living with frailty is around fifteen percent in the first month, and almost half of those admitted with a serious infection

---

[18] Bhatnagar P (2016); 'Trends in the epidemiology of cardiovascular disease in the UK'; Heart 102:1945-1952

[19] Ford E *et al* (2007); 'Explaining the decrease in US deaths from coronary disease, 1980-2000'; NEJM 356:2388-2398

[20] Cancer Research UK; www.cancerresearchuk.org/health-professional/cancer-statistics/survival/all-cancers-combined; accessed 30/12/2020

will not survive another year. In other words, strong antibiotics in such situations are often only managing to postpone the inevitable by a few months. Of course, this may be valued extra time, but we have all heard comments such as, "It was such a relief when she finally died," or, "His life was really over years ago," or indeed felt that way ourselves about a loved one. I certainly heard such comments often enough working on older people's wards.

Ageism and anti-ageing

The twentieth century movement against ageism, a term first coined in 1968, contends that one must not discriminate on the basis of age, as there is nothing distinctly different about being old. In an attempt to abolish stereotypes of ageing as useless and unproductive, the critics of ageism sought to imply that chronological age is irrelevant. This is of greatest importance to those facing retirement and who continue to seek a full, active life. We are right to consider everyone of equal value regardless of age, just as God does. But age is not irrelevant. Indeed, the COVID pandemic has shown most dramatically how those over eighty were at the greatest risk by far; the mortality rate from the infection was 0.1% in the under forties, and nearer ten percent for the over eighties. Age does change us; for instance, our immune system, our muscle fibres, our bone density, the elasticity of our skin and the number of brain cells. We are different as we age. When making decisions about the benefits and risk of an operation, age as well as the degree of frailty must be taken into account, as age always has a strong influence on the chance of success.

The origins of trying to pretend that ageing can be stopped stretch back to the mythologies of the Holy Grail. In the middle ages, the Christian view of the life course was to pursue holiness or righteousness, so that by the end of your life you were prepared for heaven. Puritans in the seventeenth century regarded your longevity to be in God's hands – a mysterious gift. They understood that old age entailed physical and mental deterioration, and pain was part of man's fallen nature.[21] Life was about a spiritual journey while accepting frailty and decline. But in the nineteenth century evangelicals would emphasise individual responsi-

---

[21] Thomas R Cole (1992); *The Journey of Life;* Cambridge University Press; see chapters 3 and 4, p.48 ff.

bility – both for salvation and the experience of your old age. If you truly cast off the old self, the new self would be strong and healthy. Victorians began to believe that hygiene and a healthy lifestyle could postpone death indefinitely. If blessed by God you would live a long life, remain vigorous and healthy and then die a natural death. The inspiration was of course derived from such Bible verses as:

> *And if you will walk in my ways, keeping my statutes and my commandments, as your father David walked, then I will lengthen your life.*[22]

> *Grey hair is a crown of glory; it is gained in a righteous life.*[23]

The corollary was that if you failed to pursue righteousness, and lived a sinful life, then you would develop disease and infirmity, and die young.

> *The fear of the LORD prolongs life, but the years of the wicked will be short.*[24]

Through the twentieth century, trust shifted from a righteous life to science as the means to postpone ageing. Now our society worships youthfulness and vitality. There is a huge anti-ageing industry spanning cosmetics, touch-up surgery and Botox – yes, our skin does rather give the game away. There are those who believe ageing can be stopped: Jean Carper's 1995 book *Stop Ageing Now!*[25] has two hundred pages describing how antioxidant vitamins, minerals, herbs and food chemicals are the magic youth potions humans have been seeking for centuries. More recently, the biologist Andrew Steele describes in his book *Ageless*[26] how ageing may be stopped; he proposes that old age is just another disease which could be prevented if enough research effort were applied.

It is hard for us to believe we will not always be here; the writer of Ecclesiastes said that God "has also set eternity in the human heart"[27]. Is this because we were made in the image of God, with God's intention

---

[22] 1 Kings 3:14 (NRSV)
[23] Proverbs 16:31 (NRSV)
[24] Proverbs 10:27 (NRSV)
[25] Carper J (1995); *Stop Ageing Now;* Harper Collins Publishers
[26] Andrew Steele (2020); *Ageless;* Bloomsbury Publishing
[27] Ecclesiastes 3:11 (NIV)

that we would live in the Garden of Eden, eating from the tree of life? Is this also why we seek immortality?

But is extreme longevity desirable? Literature contains some stark warnings: Jonathan Swift tells of Gulliver meeting the immortal Struldbruggs who were a frightening sight in their infirmities; and in Greek mythology the goddess Eos marries the mortal Tithonus, and confers on him immortality but without eternal youth – Tithonus ages and shrivels up, ultimately becoming an immortal grasshopper!

We could understand the place of modern medicine in advancing old age better if we developed a balanced and realistic view of ageing. Muriel Gillick, an American geriatrician, in her excellent 2007 book *The Denial of Ageing*[28], said:

> *We don't want to think about ageing because the prospect of losing bodily integrity, giving up our much-prized in-dependence, and nearing the end of life's journey is terrifying to us. We tend to regard old age as hopelessly, irredeemably awful, and the only way we have come up with for dispelling this view is to try to transform it into its opposite – a period that is at once deeply fulfilling and endlessly entertaining. The truth is far more complex, textured and fraught with possibility.*

I joked at the start of this chapter about just when do we become 'geriatric'? It is better to think not of a particular age, but rather when our physical abilities are changing and making us more vulnerable. Geriatricians call this frailty.

For you to consider

- What surprised you most to learn in this chapter?
- Do you sometimes think of living for ever? Can you imagine not being here?
- Do you believe that Jesus offers eternal life?

---

[28] THE DENIAL OF AGEING: PERPETUAL YOUTH, ETERNAL LIFE, AND OTHER DANGEROUS FANTASIES by Muriel R. Gillick, M.D., Cambridge, Mass.: Harvard University Press, Copyright © 2006 by the President and Fellows of Harvard College.

Chapter Two

Living With Frailty

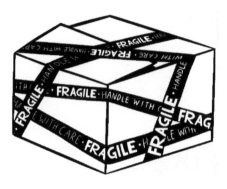

I will be your God throughout your lifetime until your hair is white with age. I made you, and I will care for you. I will carry you along and save you.[29]

IT WAS PROBABLY NO SURPRISE THAT I FOUND MY CAREER IN medicine – I was following in the footsteps of my sister, father, grandfather and great-grandfather. After four generations of GPs in Edinburgh, it was more of a surprise for me to move into hospital medicine. The attraction of geriatrics was being a 'GP' for older people in the hospital. Geriatrics was a Cinderella specialty then, and its patients often ridiculed. But in truth, working with older people has been immensely rewarding for me, partly because there was almost always something very tangible my team and I could do to help, and partly because older people are so grateful for the time and attention given to them.

Nobody wants to be labelled as being 'frail'. The word conjures up a deep fear of losing independence, dignity and control over one's life. A report by Age UK followed interviews with older people in attempting to

---

[29] Isaiah 46:4 (NLT)

understand what they felt about the concept of frailty. Here are some extracts from this report:

> *The word 'frailty' was understood to mean an irreversible state that some older people enter into in the very final stages of their lives. It was assumed that frailty means an almost total loss of independence, and there was no sense that frailty exists on a spectrum or is a state that one can move in and out of ... Beliefs were that many elements of frailty are an inevitable or unavoidable part of ageing, but that losing your independence is not.*
>
> *By contrast, the experience of living with frailty is understood as comprising a number of specific challenges and specific solutions. When older people begin to find everyday tasks harder to complete, their first instinct tends to be to find their own solutions – Medical professionals are not seen by older people as the first port of call for receiving help with everyday challenges. Older people tended to be quite proud of the coping mechanisms that they had devised for themselves. Once they move past a certain 'trigger point', however, some older people then become much more open to external support.[30]*

Ingenious solutions

As a geriatrician, I often visited people in their own homes, and came across many inventive solutions to the challenges faced by those growing old: an array of old furniture positioned to enable a slightly safer traverse around the room; ingenuity around new uses for a walking frame; and inventive seat raisers from an assortment of books and magazines. Many of these 'solutions' centred around bodily functions and toileting: the use of different pieces of clothing or newspapers to catch urine; buckets and pans as commodes; and probably the worst was finding piles of newspaper-wrapped faeces in the back kitchen, as the only toilet was blocked. Solutions to a decaying home were also common – I will never

---

[30] Age UK (2015); 'Frailty: language and perceptions'; https://www.ageuk.org.uk/globalassets/age-uk/documents/reports-and-publications/reports-and-briefings/health--wellbeing/rb_june15_frailty_language_and_perceptions.pdf

forget the somewhat eccentric eighty-five-year-old man who was rescued from his country manor roof where he had been attempting to repair a leaking roof by replacing some broken tiles. Luckily, his shouting attracted the attention of a passer-by in an adjacent field! Did any of those patients regard themselves as frail? The transition from 'battling on and just about coping' into 'struggling and feeling frustrated' is a potential moment when someone might accept they are becoming a little frail and more open to the idea of help.

Frailty is loss of reserve

Frailty is a key concept which underpins everything I am saying in this book. 'Frail' has the same linguistic root as 'fragile', derived from the Latin *fragilis*, meaning 'easily broken'. The Archbishop of Canterbury, Justin Welby, said in his 2021 New Year's message how the year of COVID "has shown us how fragile we are; it has also shown us how to face that fragility". Likewise, we need to face our frailty; as the psalmist says, "So teach us to number our days that we may gain a heart of wisdom."[31]

From a medical perspective, frailty is both distinct from age – there are very old people who are definitely not frail – and distinct from disability – there are young people who through an accident or illness have acquired a disability but are certainly not frail. The mechanism underlying frailty is a progressive loss of 'reserve' in our organs. The speed that we lose reserve varies from person to person, and indeed from organ to organ. However, almost everyone loses bone density as we age, risking broken fragile bones, and almost everyone loses muscle, leading to weakness and slowing up. Other processes may be more hidden such as loss of kidney function or lung capacity. All our organs are built with considerable reserve – for example, our pancreas will only develop diabetes when we lose over eighty percent of pancreatic capacity; Parkinson's disease will be spotted only when we have lost eighty percent of the dopamine-producing nerve cells in our brain. The built-in reserve we all have provides a degree of safety margin for the organ's function.

The loss of reserve goes unnoticed until an exceptional demand is made on that organ. For example, if we only ever walk at a gentle pace and then suddenly try to run twenty yards for a bus, we may find our

---

[31] Psalm 90:12(NIV)

muscles are weak and we have no puff left, yet we considered ourself to be fairly normal. The limited reserve in our heart, lungs and muscles is now all too obvious. Loss of reserve in the immune system results in susceptibility to infection; loss of reserve in the brain might result in acute confusion when we are ill from a simple infection; loss of reserve in the kidneys might result in kidney failure after a course of antibiotics or blood pressure pills.

So, there is a rather wide gulf between the medical view of frailty – weakness and widespread loss of reserve – and what older people themselves think – a total loss of independence. Doctors see frailty as a process akin to ageing, which for many years goes by hardly noticed as reserve is steadily lost, but then perhaps a crisis occurs – a fall, an illness, a course of medicines or an admission to hospital. The crisis stresses our body and calls upon our reserves. If reserves are insufficient, independence may be lost, and there is a temporary need for care from others at home or in hospital, followed by a time of recovery hopefully back to independence again. But perhaps recovery takes rather longer each time and is more of a struggle because there is less reserve to call upon. That experience exposes the underlying ageing process that doctors call frailty.

So how common is frailty?

While there is no universal agreement on when we become 'frail', the largest English study found frailty in twelve percent of seventy- to seventy-nine-year-olds, thirty percent of eighty- to eighty-nine-year-olds and sixty-five percent of those over ninety years.[32] And there are degrees of frailty: in the UK, the estimates are that fifty percent of older people are 'fit' or free from frailty, thirty-five percent have mild frailty, twelve percent have moderate frailty and three percent have severe frailty. And unless a sudden illness comes along, worsening frailty occurs quite slowly. The change from mild frailty to moderate frailty takes on average three years, and the change from moderate to severe frailty develops over two years.

---

[32] Gale, C *et al* (2015); 'Prevalence of frailty and disability: findings from the English Longitudinal Study of Ageing'; Age Ageing 44:162-5

Why is this important?

Recognising we are becoming frail needs to change our perspectives on life. Consider it God's warning sign that life is moving on, especially to those who have never thought about what happens after death. Chronological age and degree of frailty combine to give the strongest predictors of years of life remaining. So it means making the most of our time, doing the things that are important to us as much as we are able, and perhaps making a will and talking to our family about such things. Accepting the start of frailty does not mean life is over or giving up on independent living. But it does mean thinking about the future. Even the ageing warrior David, a biblical hero, had to accept that his warring days were over after he was cornered, nearly killed and then rescued in a battle with the Philistines. His men then declared, "Never again will you go out with us to battle."[33] Nevertheless, David was still King.

A little later, when David was "very old, no matter how many blankets covered him, he could not keep warm"[34]. Clearly a sign of frailty, but perhaps the modern equivalent is thinking about where we live – would our home be adaptable should our walking get more difficult? My mother-in-law had an old solid-fuel central heating system requiring fuel to be shovelled in almost daily (how she didn't fall more often, I have no idea), and I have often visited others tending coal fires, all at considerable risk. It felt like hitting your head against a brick wall to persuade her to invest in a new boiler – though we did get as far as having some estimates! Being able to get into and around our house, and having accessible toilets and washing facilities on the ground floor, can make all the difference to being able to continue at home after a severe illness. But inertia to do anything can be overwhelming. So many people find it too difficult to contemplate spending money on a key adaptation such as a downstairs toilet or a wet-room shower with seat. There is comfort in familiarity, while change is threatening. And those who have lived through the war learnt how to 'make do'. Yet these modest changes to the home can make an enormous difference to being able to stay at home with reduced risk. This was recently proven in research from Wales;[35] in those with moderate or severe frailty, their study showed a

---

[33] 2 Samuel 21:17 (NIV)
[34] 1 Kings 1:1 (NLT)
[35] Hollinghurst J *et al* (2020); 'Do home modifications reduce care home admissions for older people?'; Age Ageing 49:1056-61

halving of the risk of admission into care both one year and three years after the home improvements. We can request a visit from an occupational therapist to consider what adaptations could be made. In the next chapter I will describe the work of community matrons, with their gift of persuasion.

What about moving home? For many there are no choices, due to poverty: over a fifth of those over seventy-five years currently live in non-decent homes which threaten their health, and thirty-nine percent have inadequate thermal comfort.[36] Home improvements to upgrade the home to 'decent' cost an average of only £4,500 and can be facilitated through grants. Care and Repair England, or a local Home Improvement Agency, are the best places to seek advice. When finance does enable choices and we have realised our home would not suit living on one floor, then moving home in the early stages of frailty is a good idea. We may consider moving nearer to our family, but need to check with them first! There is a large supply of retirement homes now, but they can be expensive to buy, and finance may determine our options.

With a realisation that we are living with frailty, perspectives on healthcare need to start changing too. Risks of falling and going to hospital are greater, and those risks can be reduced with simple things: wearing correct glasses and some good shoes, and a having a little less clutter around. Healthcare itself also carries greater risks, such as our pills, an operation or a stay in hospital. We will look at these things later. As frailty progresses, our horizon comes closer – what can be done to help us now, not in some years' time? Frailty brings with it an increased risk of a sudden illness. We might begin thinking ahead with our friends and family, who might be able to help us through a time of need. A 'crisis back-up plan' would be a great idea, ready to swing into action – who will look after the house, the dog or the cat if we were in hospital? Who might be able to help with meals and shopping?

Frailty flags

If we are still unsure whether we, or someone we care for, is now living with frailty, here are some practical flags, any one of which might be a sign:

---

[36] Centre for Ageing Better (2020); Home-and-dry-report.pdf; ageing-better.org.uk

- Our walking has slowed up and we need to use a walking aid inside, rarely going out of the house now. We struggle on the stairs. We use a Zimmer frame!
- We have had a couple of falls while doing nothing out of the ordinary: "I was just going to answer the bell..."; "I was just going through to the kitchen when..."
- When we were last ill, we needed help from others until we recovered.
- Our GP reviewed our pills recently and stopped some of our pills as they were doing us more harm than good.
- We have never really recovered since a hospital admission this year.
- We are needing help every day with looking after ourselves.

Can frailty be stopped or reversed?

When frailty is identified, the best advice is to have a thorough review – this is explained in the next chapter. This might identify treatable conditions, as well as sorting out all sorts of problems. Making regular use of any recommended walking aid and hearing aid may mean swallowing some pride ("Don't shout, I can hear you perfectly!") but makes sense. Having bought a hearing aid that is easy to use, it needs to be worn daily for the brain to adjust to it. But good hearing is so important for maintaining social connections. According to research, the best advice to slow the frailty process is to take exercise and eat more protein. Exercise for those in their eighties and nineties need not be arduous but must be regular and maintained; twenty minutes each day of exercises to improve strength and balance is effective.[37] Tai Chi and Pilates are both excellent, although this needs motivation, and a physical ability that will be beyond many. For those less able, just walking and going up and down the stairs may be the best that can be achieved to help slow the deterioration.

In terms of nutrition, eating enough is the most important thing, particularly for those who are already underweight. Extra protein seems to be the best thing, rather than more cake and sweets often favoured by

---

[37] Kidd T (2019); 'What are the most effective interventions to improve physical performance in pre-frail and frail adults? A systematic review of randomised control trials'; BMC Geriatrics 19:184

some older people. Taste buds become less sensitive as we age, needing stronger saltiness or sweetness, which, combined with reduced sense of smell, makes meals less appetising. Some extra spice or salt can help. Most vitamin supplements are harmless but unnecessary for almost everyone, although a vitamin D supplement is recommended if confined to the house. Most diabetics, apart from those who have had a lifetime of insulin, need not worry about sticking to any diet now – just eat a little more protein.

Finding value in the Fourth Age

The Third Age is the extended period of retirement most of us are able to enjoy. The period of reduced independence towards the end of life which the majority of us will experience might be termed the Fourth Age. The current generation living in the Fourth Age could be termed pioneers, as in the past only the few would live into their nineties. Can there be value and purpose during these years of disability, when we are no longer productive?

Ancient literature almost exclusively emphasised a negative view of old age, often linked to evil and witches. In ancient Greek literature youth was generally sweet, beautiful and heroic; old age was ugly, mean and tragic. The Old Testament, by contrast, has a much more positive view on the mutual strengths of vigour in the young and wisdom in the old. "The glory of young men is their strength, but the splendour of old men is their grey hair."[38] The New Testament has some of the most beautiful illustrations of the value God places on old age, recorded by Luke the physician:

- Elizabeth, pregnant with John in her old age, was the first to acknowledge the presence of Christ in Mary's womb.[39]
- Simeon had been promised by God that he would not die before seeing the Christ and waited in faithfulness.[40]
- Anna, an eighty-four-year-old widow, continued to serve God in the temple, worshipping day and night and recognised the divinity

---

[38] Proverbs 20:29 (ESV)
[39] Luke 1:41
[40] Luke 2:25-26

of Christ, witnessing the fact to all around.[41] Clearly there is no retirement from God's work for Christians.

- Jesus acknowledges the sacrificial giving of the widow who "out of her poverty put in all she had to live on"[42].

The psalmist says, "They still bear fruit in old age..."[43] This may be influenced by the severity of disability and any mental disorder such as dementia. "The truth is far more complex, textured and fraught with possibility"[44] as Dr Gillick said in the previous chapter. There is a wealth of Christian literature to encourage us: try David Winter's *At the End of the Day*[45] or Ian Knox's *Finishing Well*[46]. But here are some simple suggestions which I have observed improve well-being and give purpose:

- *Remembrance and reflection*
  When we are no longer able to do so much, there is time on our hands. We can reflect on our life and try to understand its legacy, if we were kept too busy in our Third Age to do this. We may wish to share our thoughts with our close family, or perhaps record memoirs.

- *Intergenerational connections*
  There have recently been wonderful examples of forming links between children in nurseries and schools with residents of care homes, which have been mutually beneficial, educational and inspiring. Similarly, such connections can be made within church congregations and their neighbourhood. Naomi's care for Ruth, and Ruth's commitment and loyalty to Naomi, is a biblical example we can follow. "O God, from my youth you have taught me, and I still proclaim your wondrous deeds. So even to old age and grey hairs, O God, do not forsake me, until I proclaim your might to another generation, your power to all those to come."[47]

---

[41] Luke 2:36-38
[42] Luke 21:4 (NIV)
[43] Psalm 92:14 (NIV)
[44] THE DENIAL OF AGEING: PERPETUAL YOUTH, ETERNAL LIFE, AND OTHER DANGEROUS FANTASIES by Muriel R. Gillick, M.D., Cambridge, Mass.: Harvard University Press, Copyright © 2006 by the President and Fellows of Harvard College.
[45] David Winter (2013); *At the End of the Day;* Bible Reading Fellowship
[46] Ian Knox (2020); *Finishing Well;* SPCK
[47] Psalm 71:17-18 (ESV)

- *Creativity*

  This may be a time for our God-inspired creativity – writing a poem or novel, artwork, knitting or sewing crafts, or music. Some of the most remarkable works of art and literature were composed in the last years of life. "Do not conform to the pattern of this world but be transformed by the renewing of your mind."[48] It must be better than the grumpy old man watching TV.

- *Prayer*

  Our personhood is not changed by disability, nor is God's love for us. We can become prayer warriors in intercession; in our prayers God may give us dreams which are prophetic for the church – "And your sons and your daughters will prophesy, your old men will dream dreams, your young men will see visions."[49] – dreams inspired by experiences from the past. Faithfulness in prayer can be a fantastic inspiration to the following generations.

Now let's consider more specifically how healthcare can be used wisely, and with a light touch, to enhance the experience of living with frailty.

For you to consider

- Have you thought about the Third Age and Fourth Age, and where you might live in your Fourth Age?
- What fears do you have for living in the Fourth Age?
- Do you recognise frailty in yourself, or your relative?
- What could you do to slow your loss of reserve?
- How will you stay fruitful in the Fourth Age? How will you strengthen your faith?

---

[48] Romans 12:2 (NIV)
[49] Joel 2:28 (NIV)

CHAPTER THREE

A Pill for All Ills?

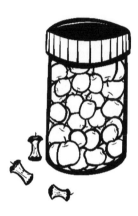

Listen to your father who gave you life, and do not despise your mother when she is old.[50]

HEALTHCARE HAS MOVED ON A LONG WAY FROM THE LATE nineteenth century aphorism, "An apple a day keeps the doctor away." Now there is not only a pill for everything, but it is increasingly common to be taking a large number of different tablets. Ray Kurzweil and Terry Grosman in their book *Transcend*[51] believed that immortality may be achievable through a combination of the correct diet and pills; Kurzweil reputedly took between 180 and 250 pills a day! Most people are doing their best to follow their doctor's orders, and pills just keep multiplying. Remembering to take all those pills at the right time can be quite a challenge – indeed around fifty percent of prescriptions are not taken exactly as intended by the prescribing doctor.

---

[50] Proverbs 23:22 (ESV)
[51] Kurzweil R, Grossman T (2010); *Transcend: Nine Steps to Living Well Forever;* Rodale Press

Offering to help with someone else's medication may receive a guarded response as if it is an attack on their independence. By contrast, I have observed some couples taking a mix-and-match approach as they borrow from each other's pills as needed! As a relative, it may have been when you started collecting the prescription from the chemist that you realised just how many pills were being taken. It can be a nightmare to follow all the different instructions, and when you start reading all the leaflets, you get even more worried. Yet we may feel our health, or the health of our relative, depends upon taking all those pills correctly. Does she really need them all? If she actually took all those pills as prescribed, might this lead to further problems? So, you consider getting more involved.

Before we explore how to review all those pills, let's consider the challenges of getting involved at all. In her book *If It's Not Too Much Trouble – The Challenge of the Aged Parent*, Ann Benton has amusing and practical advice for Christians seeking to care for their parents derived from her own experience.[52] She describes the common, but so true, coping mechanisms that older people may use when dealing with others:

- *Fussiness*
  "Why can't you just get the ones I like? Just leave it there."
- *Self-pity*
  "No-one understands what it's like; no-one listens."
- *Anger*
  "You never come to see me. Why isn't it any better by now?"
- *Denial*
  "I'm fine. I'll do it my way; I like it this way."
- *Dependence*
  "It's alright, my daughter will do it for me; you're not going already?"
- *Martyrdom*
  "Don't you bother about me; you have your life. You can phone tomorrow if I am still here."

I think my wife and I have observed most of these in her mother over the last year, and some in relation to pills and potions. These mechanisms

---

[52] Ann Benton (2007); *If It's Not Too Much Trouble – The Challenge of the Aged Parent;* Christian Focus

may be deeply ingrained, and perhaps shaped by a person's life experiences over many years, as well as their innate personality. Personality traits often seem to become exaggerated as we age – a warning there! If we think we are being drawn into the caring role, we will undoubtedly need to rely on God's enabling strength and the fruit of the Spirit in abundance. We might find repeating the words of the Grace of value:[53]

- *"May the grace of our Lord Jesus Christ..."*
  The grace to forgive the fussiness, anger or stoicism thrown at us.
- *"...the love of God..."*
  The love to listen patiently, to speak the honest truth and to explain why it is this way.
- *"...the fellowship of the Holy Spirit..."*
  The fruit of the Spirit to sustain us, and the grace to accept fellowship and support from others.

Sometimes the community matrons may be called upon to solve a medication puzzle like Simon's.

Simon was only sixty-two years old when he was referred to the local community matron because almost every week he was being admitted to hospital as an emergency with a hypoglycaemic attack – a low blood sugar. The GP was desperate to find a way to stop this happening. He was known to have a number of diseases which included diabetes, COPD (a form of chronic lung disease) and coronary artery disease. The community matron visited him at home, where he lived alone. She found a year's worth of medication scattered throughout the flat in multiple cupboards, drawers and boxes, and a non-working fridge!

I will explain a little later how the community matron found some solutions.

---

[53] 2 Corinthians 13:14 (NIV)

A mountain of pills

The increase in medicine use in the UK has been quite dramatic in the last twenty years or so. A large UK study of older people living at home[54] compared figures from 1991 with 2008. In 1991 the most common number of medicines was two and the most for any individual was eight; in 2008 this had increased to an average of five and a maximum of twenty-three. The proportion of people on five or more medicines had increased from twelve to fifty percent, and in the over seventy-fives it had reached sixty percent. It is likely the numbers are even higher now. Those on no medicines had dropped from twenty percent to eight percent.

A recent review found that one in three older people are taking a pill that could be harming them.[55] That study reckoned that within a population of older people at home, harms from medicines could be responsible for as many as one in six attendances at an emergency department and eleven percent of unplanned hospital admissions.

Because of this, it has become important for those living with frailty to have a regular thorough review of medications. The process is also referred to as 'deprescribing', as a common beneficial result is reducing the overall number of medicines being taken. Too much of a good thing can make us worse. It is astonishing just how much better one can feel when told to take fewer tablets. Before having a discussion with the doctor, see how far you can understand the following steps. (These steps are derived from the NHS Scotland publication on polypharmacy.[56])

Step one: Understand current medicines

In my experience most older people have only the vaguest notion of the purpose of many of their pills, but they usually do know the painkillers and the bowel medicines. This shows which pills they regard as important. My heart would sink when I asked to see the medicines someone was taking and a large box or carrier bag containing assorted blister packs was tipped out onto the desk. It started to resemble a pick-and-mix! It is hard to judge whether a pill is effective if we are unsure

---

[54] Gao L *et al* (2018); 'Medication usage change in older people (65+) in England over 20 years: findings from CFASI and CFAS II'; Age and Ageing, Volume 47, Issue 2, March 2018; pp.220-225

[55] Age UK (2019); 'More harm than good'

[56] Polypharmacy-Guidance-2018.pdf; scot.nhs.uk

what it is trying to achieve. Sometimes, a member of the family had written out, or typed up, a chart to indicate the purpose of that tablet and when each was to be taken. The patient might proudly produce this list, confirming its value in their eyes – and also to me. See if you can make such a chart.

Step two: Identify which pills are most important

Some pills are only effective and safe if taken reliably every day, and pills vary in their importance for an individual. For example, thyroxine for someone with thyroid deficiency, or hydrocortisone for someone with adrenal gland deficiency, is essential and even lifesaving. So, we need to know which pills are essential. The doctor can clarify this if we are unsure.

RELIEVERS

The rest of our medication can generally be divided into those which are symptom remedies ('relievers'), and those which are trying to prevent some disease ('preventers') or a worsening of an existing disease in the future. The symptom relievers are, for example, painkillers, sleeping tablets, treatments for indigestion and simple bowel disorders, and some angina tablets. For some people who really need those tablets, then missing them for a few days will quickly lead to the symptoms worsening. For others, the symptom relievers can be taken as and when needed; the advantage here is reducing the overall number of pills we need to take every day and thereby reducing side-effects. For these reliever pills, it is acceptable to try a few days without that pill to know whether indeed it must be taken every day or just from time to time.

A special note about painkillers. Pain is experienced by almost everyone who lives with frailty, and it is difficult to treat without side-effects and even more difficult to abolish. Thankfully, some of us have high pain thresholds so we notice it less than others. Physiotherapy and nerve stimulation devices can be enormously helpful and avoid the side-effects of pills. Regular use of painkillers is better than intermittent use, and may well help preserve independence and mobility, even if the pain does not go away completely. Painkiller patches are useful to give continuous pain relief – especially for someone who might forget to take the tablets regularly. The side-effect of constipation can be sorted as needed, but too strong painkillers can easily upset balance or cause confusion. Good advice from our doctor is needed.

PREVENTERS

Most other medication is a 'preventer' – trying to reduce something happening in the future. Some of the most common preventers are:

- aspirin to prevent a heart attack;
- a statin to prevent all types of circulatory disease;
- tablets to lower blood pressure to reduce heart disease, strokes and kidney failure;
- diabetic tablets to prevent kidney failure and circulatory disease;
- and anticoagulants to prevent strokes.

In these situations, the pills work on a statistical or probability basis: if one hundred people take pill Y for two years, then compared with one hundred who don't take pill Y, there will be, say, five fewer strokes. For those five people, the pill has been a success, while the other ninety-five have taken the pill with no apparent benefit to them. Of course, the doctor cannot know who the five lucky ones are who will avoid the stroke – that is a lottery. This is known as the 'number needed to treat' – or NNT. So, for pill Y the NNT is twenty for two years – twenty people need to take the treatment for two years for one person to benefit through an avoided event. This may be expressed as two years, because that is how long the treatment needs to be taken before it starts to give real benefit. Doctors will generally know, based on research, how long it takes before a particular treatment becomes effective. For those with advancing frailty who may be nearing the end of life, a treatment that takes several years to be of benefit may not be considered worthwhile.

WHAT ABOUT TARGETS?

We may be familiar with the idea of a target for a certain pill. For example, our GP says we have not reached our target blood pressure, so we need an extra pill or a higher dose of the current one; or our cholesterol is still above the target, so again we need a higher dose of the statin. Targets need to be different for people living with frailty. In fact, there is quite a problem if the familiar targets from guidelines are applied directly to older people living with frailty. The usual target is based on getting the right balance between the beneficial effect and minimising the side-effects, derived from research studies. For diabetes, for example, the target figure for the blood test is higher in those living with frailty, because they have a higher risk of hypoglycaemia (a low blood sugar as a side-effect) and less chance of benefiting from good diabetic control, because the benefits take five to ten years to be seen. Similarly, for blood pressure, the best balance between benefit and side-effects is to have a blood pressure around 150 mmHg. Those with this blood pressure live the longest. This will seem rather high to younger people on blood pressure pills. Hence the importance of regular review of our medicines, as the targets change as our health changes.

COMPETING RISKS

Unfortunately, it is difficult to know if preventers are of similar value to those living with frailty as to those who are more able. As mentioned before, the studies which have measured the benefit have been with younger people or able-bodied older people. In addition, the benefits may not be as good as hoped because of what is known as 'competing risks' – or the law of diminishing returns. Someone with frailty will probably have multiple pills and several different conditions. Several pills may each have the same aim of, say, reducing a stroke, but taken together the benefit is less than the sum of the parts. For instance, the pill for blood pressure may reduce the risk by a quarter, and the pill for irregular heartbeat reduces the risk also by a quarter, but when taken together the pills do not halve the risk of stroke – the benefit turns out to be rather less. And, apart from this, the person's health or life expectancy may be determined more by a different disease altogether. So, all in all, the benefits of the preventer pills are more difficult to judge, and understanding our priorities for prevention is helpful to the doctor in choosing wisely.

Step three: Identify unnecessary medications

Following step two, it will become clear if some pills can be taken occasionally rather than regularly. Indeed, if the symptoms have stopped, the pill may now not be needed at all. For some pills, the objective of the treatment may no longer be important. For example, the pill to prevent angina is probably unnecessary if we are no longer able to walk or exert ourselves; or the pill to prevent seizures is unnecessary if there have been no seizures for many years.

Almost invariably I would find one or more medications which had been prescribed to treat the side-effects of another pill, creating a sort of medicine escalator. It would be preferable to stop both medications if possible – the one causing the side-effect as well as the one treating the side-effect. It may well be difficult to unravel the reason for the medications and the sequence of events without going through this with a doctor.

If a medication review takes place at home, or if family members continue the process back at home, there may be some interesting revelations of medicines no longer used or out-of-date. When I was reviewing my mother-in-law's medicines prior to her moving into a residential care home, we discovered not only the Tupperware box with her current prescriptions, but also two drawers and one shelf full of boxes and medicines dating back many years. My wife was delighted to hand four large carrier bags into the local chemist – he was not so delighted to receive them!

LIVING WITH SEVERE FRAILTY

For those whose life is much more limited, perhaps now largely confined to bed or living in a nursing home, or possibly in the last year of life, medications trying to prevent things will seem to be rather irrelevant. For them, the important thing is comfort and quality of life. One of the benefits of identifying severe frailty, or the likelihood of being in the last year of life, is that the burden of multiple pills can be cut back considerably. For them, targets are irrelevant. Control of symptoms has become the most important thing.

Step four: Are the current treatments effective?

For some pills, a review may establish that the pill has never achieved its purpose – a painkiller, an antidepressant, a sleeping tablet or a bladder pill that gave no improvement to the symptom. The pill may well have been started as a trial to see if it would help but was never reviewed. The reason for the treatment not working could include it was not taken sufficiently often or regularly, or at the right dosage. But of course, equally it may be the treatment was just not effective for the symptom or problem.

For the preventer pills, judging whether the pill is achieving its purpose is more difficult. It may be possible to see that seizures or asthma attacks have been reduced. But for others, just not having another stroke or not breaking a bone must be taken as success, although it is impossible to know if that is because of the medication or just good fortune. But when an event like that happens, it should lead to a doctor reviewing to see if the treatments can be improved upon.

Step five: Are there risks of adverse drug reactions?

Unfortunately, as people age, the risk of side-effects with each medicine increases. This is true for almost every medicine and is partly because the reduced reserve in our organs inherent in frailty alters the ability of our body to make the necessary adjustments to handle the new drug safely. For almost every tablet, there is a risk that the medicine could actually do more harm than good, and this becomes much more evenly balanced than for most younger people. In simple terms, the more tablets we take, the greater the likelihood of side-effects. Some side-effects might hardly be noticed, while others could be serious enough to lead to an emergency hospital admission. And we shouldn't be fooled just because we have taken a tablet for many years without any problems – ageing and the impact of frailty could easily mean that this familiar tablet is now no longer safe for us.

The simplest way of reducing the risk of adverse effects is just to take fewer medicines. A medication review in someone with frailty will usually come up with some tablets no longer useful because the symptoms are less, or because the tablet has not proved to be effective. Some medications combine to heighten the side-effect problem – for example, side-effects such as dizziness, tiredness, dry mouth or falling. So just taking fewer of the tablets that give a similar side-effect can be helpful. Identifying the tablets of least value (from step two) helps decide which tablets might now be dropped to improve the side-effect problem.

Will the plan be stuck to?

By the end of this process and discussion with our doctor, we should have a clear plan about what treatment is to be taken and what is being stopped. Hopefully, we have agreed with this plan and understand the reasons for making changes. A written reminder card describing when to take each tablet can be extremely useful when a lot of tablets are involved. This may also need to be rewritten after a hospital admission or clinic. The chemist may issue the tablets in a weekly tray if the GP agrees this would help. There is one gadget which emits a beep or even speaks a recorded message as a reminder that tablets are due, and then a container pops open.

But sometimes we may be reluctant to stop taking a tablet or medicine taken faithfully for many years, with fear of an old problem returning. While stopping the medicine might have been agreed in front of the doctor, we have a change of heart once back home. And perhaps we remember that years ago a doctor said to take this tablet "for the rest of your life". The plan will no doubt require adjusting in the weeks and months ahead, so some of the changes can be viewed as a trial, but the potential reward of fewer medicines is worthwhile.

Don't rock the boat

The doctor or nurse carrying out the medication review may also have anxieties about withdrawing medication. This can stem from a fear of 'rocking the boat' if our health is reasonably stable at present and risking triggering further problems. In reducing medications, the doctor does not wish to give the impression that they are giving up on us – "You're not worth these tablets anymore." But the truth is quite the opposite. In my experience, most people are only too delighted to take fewer medicines. There can be encouragement – "Look, Mum, the doctor says you don't these now." Some will feel better just because they do not need to take so many pills. Because of the cumulative effect of multiple medications on the body, there can often be improved well-being and energy from the reduced burden of medication.

Community matrons and comprehensive reviews

Let's return to the story about Simon and his repeated admissions to hospital.

After several long chats, Simon revealed to the community matron that he could not read and did not recognise numbers, therefore guessed all medication and doses. Over a period of months, the matron worked with Simon, gaining his confidence and agreement to make some changes. First, a pill dispenser with verbal prompts was put in place to tell him when to take his tablets. The community diabetic team provided pictorial advice cards and a talking glucometer that records the blood sugar level. The matron contacted social care, who provided support with shopping to ensure there was fresh food in the house – and hopefully towards a healthier diet. The housing support officer assisted with making the flat safer, and a local charity provided a working fridge.

Simon had slipped through the safety net as he was ashamed about not being able to read and had been labelled a 'time waster' as no one had ever asked why he struggled to care for himself. Given the right support he has not had any further admissions due to hypoglycaemia and feels more confident in caring for himself. He has now agreed to ongoing support to help him with literacy.

The NHS and social care are under such pressure, and the demands of frail older people on the health and social care system are so overwhelming, that in recent years a proactive initiative has emerged to identify and support people living with frailty. We might reasonably think that the GP would already be aware of all their patients living with frailty. In this country people see their GP or practice nurse on average five times a year, but older people consult far more often: for those between sixty-five and seventy-four it is eight times a year; between seventy-five and eighty-four it is eleven times; and for those over eighty-five it is thirteen times.[57] But most of these visits are limited by the consulting time available from the GP, which is about ten minutes, as we all know. As older people will have several long term conditions and potentially multiple issues they could talk about, it is not surprising that this is difficult and stressful for everyone. A study from the University of Bristol[58] found that an average consultation included discussion of 2.5 different problems across a wide range of disease areas in less than twelve minutes, with each additional problem being discussed in just two minutes. There are other factors also at play which may hold back those living with frailty from seeking help – embarrassment of admitting to the problems or fear of being forced into a care home, for example. In addition, anyone with dementia may not have the insight to appreciate their need of help.

---

[57] www.kingsfund.org.uk/sites/default/files/field/field_publication_file/ Understanding-GP-pressures-Kings-Fund-May-2016.pdf; accessed 30/12/2020

[58] Salisbury C *et al* (2013); 'The content of general practice consultations: cross-sectional study based on video recordings'; British Journal of General Practice, Volume 63, no.616, e751-9

Frailty assessments

Primary care is now encouraged to identify proactively all those living with frailty and arrange a thorough assessment of their problems and needs. This is with the hope that doing so will not only be appreciated, but also reduce the chance of more intractable problems further downstream. The assessment for frailty is often carried out by a community nurse or community matron and is called 'comprehensive geriatric assessment' (CGA). This cumbersome title is clearly not very age-friendly, and an Age UK report[59] found that older people, and indeed many healthcare staff, struggle to understand what it means.

> *...older people were concerned about how long the assessment would take, which specialists they would see, and what effort would be required on their part. These concerns were especially true of older people who were already managing serious health conditions and who said that they wanted to avoid further 'hassle' and medical intervention in their lives.*

They suggested it might be called "the over 75's MOT" – but it is actually offered to those with frailty, regardless of age. CGA is a programme of assessment, treatment and monitoring which has been shown to benefit those living with frailty and might slow the progression into greater dependency.[60] The British Geriatric Society recently published a thorough guide for Primary Care in the UK on just how to deliver CGA.[61] In summary, it involves physical, functional, social and environmental assessment, mental health review and medication review; this is followed by creating an action list which leads to a care plan and subsequent monitoring of the interventions agreed. There are a growing number of specialist community nurses, some called community matrons,

---

[59] Age UK (2015); 'Frailty: language and perceptions'; https://www.ageuk.org.uk/globalassets/age-uk/documents/reports-and-publications/reports-and-briefings/health--wellbeing/rb_june15_frailty_language_and_perceptions.pdf

[60] Ekdahl A *et al* (2016); 'Long-term evaluation of the ambulatory geriatric assessment: a frailty intervention trial (AGE-FIT)'; J Am Med Dir Assoc 17(3):263-8

[61] British Geriatric Society (2019); 'Comprehensive geriatric assessment toolkit for Primary Care Practitioners'; https://www.bgs.org.uk/sites/default/files/content/resources/files/2019-03-12/CGA%20Toolkit%20for%20Primary%20Care%20Practitioners_0.pdf

who will take a person living with frailty through this process. They can be a lifeline and an advocate where prior to this the person was struggling to find their way through the maze of services. Having a community matron chat to us in our own home over a cup of tea, listening to all our problems and working out what can be done to help, might be less threatening than a visit to the GP. Where someone has had a positive experience with support services, perhaps for a small problem, they are going to be more open to support on a future occasion. Older people often feel they are up against a brick wall and a community matron could be a life saver.

Here is another illustration of how a community matron and I resolved a confusing medication problem.

TOO MUCH OF A GOOD THING

Tom was seventy-eight and a great character. He had always been 'one of the lads', enjoying socialising at the pub after work and being quite an independent spirit. He had three children by his first marriage and had been married to his present wife for over twenty years. He was always the one to make the decisions in the marriage. He had become a diabetic in his fifties and moved onto insulin in his sixties, finding it difficult to keep to his diet. He did his insulin injections twice a day and this was fine until he became forgetful. A year before I met him, he had been diagnosed as having vascular dementia, so his wife took over supervision of the insulin, although he insisted he was fine without her help. He loved walking into town where he would meet his friends at a local cafe.

The community matron asked me to see him because the GP could not understand why he kept running out of insulin before it was due. Yet his blood sugars were generally too high, not too low as might be expected if he was overdosing on insulin. Eventually the community matron and I worked out that although his wife had measured out and supervised his morning insulin injection, he would then have forgotten perhaps half an hour later and gone to the fridge and given himself another dose. Then he would feel hungry as his sugar level was dropping – so enjoyed a second breakfast in town. He was also consuming a packet of chocolate digestives most days. We had to get his wife to lock up his insulin and insist that she bought no more biscuits! His diabetic control improved thereafter – but we were never going to stop him going into town!

For you to consider

- Do you understand what each tablet is for?
- Is a medication review with your GP overdue?
- Does your GP have a linked community matron? Do you think a visit might help?

CHAPTER FOUR

A Few More Tests

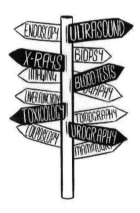

Then you will know the truth, and the truth will set you free...[62]

MARGARET LIVED IN ONE OF OUR MORE RURAL PARTS OF the county and had been a teacher all her working life – indeed a head teacher for ten years – with no close family. Her health had gradually deteriorated over the last year, losing weight and strength, but she had not bothered anyone and reckoned this was just her age. She now had become a little breathless, unsteady on her feet and housebound. She met our team at the hospital after a fall and some bruises. When we examined her, we found she was a little clumsy with her hands. Her blood test revealed anaemia and a profoundly low vitamin B12 level. When this deficiency is severe, it can cause loss of feeling in the legs as well as anaemia and could easily have been the reason for her troubles. She just needed some vitamin injections. When I saw her in the clinic the following month, she was much stronger and the breathlessness had gone, although her walking was still quite unsteady.

---

[62] John 8:32 (NIV)

The power to interrogate the human body – its working and its structure – has grown phenomenally through the advent of modern medicine. When I was taught in medical school in the 1970s, we were instructed that the patient's history would provide eighty percent of the answer, a physical examination would confirm your thoughts and suggest ideas for another ten percent, and tests would be used to confirm your hypothesis or reveal a different answer in the remaining ten percent. Most doctors would still insist that this has not changed and that careful listening holds the key to making a correct diagnosis. The investigations should follow on from this and be viewed as a way of testing the hypothesis, or perhaps just the doctor's hunch, to see if the suspected diagnosis can be confirmed.

For older people living with frailty, a blood test can be enormously helpful. Problems can creep up with none of the usual symptoms to help the doctor make the diagnosis. The only symptoms may be rather non-specific – "just not right"; "a bit weak and wobbly today"; "seem to have lost all my energy". How do you distinguish this from an off day that any of us might have? Familiarity with the person can help enormously here – judging what is different from the usual 'off day'. But the person living with frailty taking multiple medications is much more vulnerable to new problems. A simple blood test and checking temperature, pulse and blood pressure are very helpful as a first step in the medicine of older people. GPs will quite properly try to avoid unnecessary tests, and their knowledge of the person will very often be able to reach a provisional diagnosis and management plan without tests. But where there is some lingering doubt about a new illness, an extra blood test in these situations can be the answer. Some older people are like Margaret and say, "Oh, I don't want to be bothering the doctor, he has quite enough to do without seeing me; it's just my age." Conversely, a normal blood test greatly reduces the chance that there is a new disease lurking.

If you have ever accompanied an older person to a hospital clinic, I wonder what was uppermost in your mind? I suspect that a fair pro-portion of your concern was taken up with finding a parking space, finding your way to the correct clinic or department without going round in circles, and maybe needing a wheelchair if the distance was too great. Then whether the clinic was running to time, and the lack of information. And then whether you could help your relative to the toilet, hoping this did not clash with when you are called in. And then just getting home. The time and effort required for the whole expedition can be considerable. But in the middle, of course, was the appointment when you hoped to learn the truth. But would that mean more tests and more visits?

What sort of person has the disease?

Living in the eighteenth century, Sir William Osler is known as the 'father of modern medicine' for revolutionising the way in which medical education was taught during his tenure at Johns Hopkins School of Medicine in the US. One of the many catchphrases he taught was, "It's more important to know what sort of person has the disease, than what sort of disease the person has." This sentence has been a guiding principle for me as a physician and geriatrician. We know God is more concerned with the person we are than with our imperfections. Person-centred medical care means listening to the patient first to understand their concerns, their hopes and fears, and what matters most to them. With care this can lead to mutual respect, which is a wonderful starting point. In the context of assessing frailty, discerning what sort of person the patient is enables the doctor to see the whole picture and what the priorities may be for any treatments. This means some careful listening before jumping in with tests. And a whole lot of tests can stir up a hornet's nest. Let me explain.

A 'normal' blood test

"So was my blood test okay?" we ask the GP receptionist on the phone. We assume there is a simple yes or no answer. But blood tests are not as black and white as many people imagine. An illustration of the difficulty comes with the troponin blood test for angina and heart disease.

Consider the situation of Gerald, an older man in his eighties who collapsed in the night and is brought up to the emergency department. He cannot remember what happened but came round on the landing floor. He had a heart attack many years ago and seems to have been fine since then. The doctor wonders if he has had a 'silent heart attack' – that is, a heart attack without pain, as this is more common as you get older. His ECG looks normal, but the troponin blood test is markedly raised. The message gets out to his family that he has a suspected heart attack. Gerald is given emergency injections for a heart attack and kept in hospital while waiting for another troponin test. (In a true heart attack, a repeat troponin blood test a short time later will have risen further.) But the repeat test is unchanged. So, he's probably okay. He might have had a heart rhythm problem that had settled before he arrived at the hospital. He is allowed home the next day after seeing the specialist, with a heart monitor test as an outpatient.

The troponin blood test shows any injury to heart muscle. It is used to identify people who need to be in hospital for urgent heart treatment. Over the years, the test has been made more and more sensitive to reduce the risk of missing a true heart attack. The majority of abnormal results do not in fact indicate a heart attack. This is particularly true for older people living with frailty attending hospital in an emergency. Many will have an abnormal troponin level permanently, through their accumulated health conditions putting a strain on the heart. In addition, the emergency itself, perhaps a fall or collapse, will have added to that strain.

Gerald's is a common scenario and can cause much stress to everyone. The problem is the enigmatic question, "Where is the truth?" If this elderly man is asked by his family (who had been told he had a suspected heart attack and want reassurance), "So is your heart okay now?" what can he say? Yes and no – both are true, and it's not black or white. In some situations, Gerald might be asked to undergo a cardiac angiogram – an imaging test to look at his coronary arteries. Because he had a heart attack years ago, and because of his age, his heart might have caused yesterday's problem. He is unlikely to have healthy coronary arteries, but his heart has not given him any trouble for years, as far as he can tell. The angiogram will probably show disease in one or more of his coronary arteries, and the guidelines have evidence that treatment will reduce the risk of a future heart attack. So, he might be scheduled for surgery, perhaps angioplasties (non-invasive surgery) or perhaps coronary bypass grafts. But if his collapse had nothing to do with his heart, should he undergo this treatment? It does have some risks. Or come to that, should he have had the treatment years ago, if it would have reduced his risk of a future heart attack?

In practice it does not work like this, at least most of the time in the UK. A senior cardiologist will review Gerald and make his or her clinical judgement as to whether there is truly a good case for further investigations: is he likely to benefit from a heart procedure, or will the risks of the procedure outweigh that possible benefit? The decision requires judgment, the experience of the specialist and perhaps their caution; hopefully, the wishes of the patient play a part too. The guidelines represent averages and cannot include calculations about the risks and benefits for this unique person. It is hard to be certain what would be the 'safest' thing to do.

This is an illustration of how one test spirals into another, not necessarily under our control, and how this can lead to difficult decisions. Guidelines and medical pathways are a route map from symptoms through tests to a diagnosis. Tests seek to improve certainty of diagnosis. They assume that evidence-based treatments will follow. There are several problems here for those with frailty:

- the symptoms are vague, so the choice of pathway is unclear;
- further tests are of greater risk in those with frailty;
- the test results are ambiguous;
- the evidence for treatment is derived from younger people.

Medicine places its trust in those pathways, making the doctor less open to criticism, ultimately criticism in court. This tends to lead risk-averse doctors towards caution and doing extra tests. It is so much easier when patients fit into a standard pathway – but old people may not quite fit. Frailty medicine requires a different way – departing at times from 'usual care' – if we are to respect the person's tolerance for tests and minimise the burden of hospitalisation. It is a middle way between 'usual care' and 'comfort-only care'. It uses enough tests to reduce uncertainty a little, and enough medicine to have given a reasonable chance of success. Above all, it places dignity and compassion to the fore. It takes courage to act this way. We will consider this again in the next chapter.

I was often asked to review a person on the admissions ward of our hospital, or in the emergency department, by another consultant who was not a geriatrician. They would say something like, "Could you take a look at my patient, please, and see what you think – she could go for a scan, but I wonder if you think she could go home?" That consultant had the gut feeling that the sensible thing was to let her home, but the usual practice and pathway was pointing to something different. A conversation with her, and a more holistic review, would guide my decision, and we would try to find a way of managing her condition back at home. "It's more important to know what sort of person has the disease, than what sort of disease the person has."

Blood tests a first step in assessment

Blood tests can be enormously valuable in assessing an older person where the symptoms are vague, or where it is obvious that the person's heath is deteriorating yet the underlying cause is unclear. Careful interpretation of the blood tests can indicate where the chief abnormality lies and where to look for disease. Correction of a vitamin or thyroid deficiency, treating anaemia, and managing dehydration or kidney failure, are common examples which can almost always be helped and might not have been identified without blood tests. This is not 'tests for the sake of tests' but a pathway in the assessment of an older person who is struggling and perhaps entering frailty.

Another UTI?

Other body fluids can also be tested, including the urine – indeed the history of this stretches back many centuries. In the Middle Ages a doctor would reach a diagnosis using his funnel-shaped glass container called a matula to inspect the urine – its colour and any cloudiness – and also taste the urine! In those days diabetes was diagnosed by sweet-tasting urine. Urine tests today are with a plastic stick which is dipped into the urine to detect any protein, blood or sugar. It can also show chemicals which indicate the presence of bacteria.

Herein is a common problem for older people: bacteria are more frequently present in the urine as we age, but their mere presence does not indicate they are causing trouble. Just as we live with bacteria in our mouths and gut all the time, so too bacteria are present in the urine. Around a quarter of older people living with frailty will have bacteria present without that causing any symptoms – a course of antibiotics would not therefore make any difference to them. When a dipstick test shows probable bacteria, it is a common mistake to interpret this as proof of a urine infection; proof lies in the laboratory urine culture result. Thousands of 'off days' have been blamed on a 'urinary tract infection', based solely on the stick test, and treated accordingly. Much of the time this might not matter but it risks causing more harm than good in those with frailty. Antibiotics can give side-effects, and a course of antibiotics increases bacterial resistance in the body so that a future true infection is less likely to respond to conventional antibiotics.

And then a scan

When a blood test has come back abnormal, a scan of some sort is commonly arranged. Thanks to ever-improving computer processing, the quality, accuracy and speed of scans is increasing all the time. This makes it very easy to scan a large part of the body in a matter of minutes. Today, the whole body can be scanned in half an hour. This has delivered enormous benefits for rapid assessment in emergency admissions, for example after a stroke or a serious injury, as well as transforming the whole identification and management of cancers. An accurate diagnosis is reached much faster, and people are much less likely to be stuck in hospital waiting for a scan.

But there are risks of overdiagnosis with our modern-day tests. For instance, the D-dimer blood test is used as a marker for blood clots on the lung; unfortunately, it is raised in lots of conditions apart from a new blood clot, and generally rises with age. An abnormal result could make a risk-averse doctor request a lung scan, even if a blood clot diagnosis did not seem very likely. The scans are very sensitive and as well as showing when there is a serious problem, can also find tiny clots. These are too small to be of importance, yet their discovery could lead to unnecessary treatment with anticoagulants for months.

Another sequence of tests is on the prostate. Here a raised prostate-specific antigen, referred to as 'PSA', can lead to a prostate scan and then biopsies. Tiny prostate tumours are common and for those living with frailty are of little significance as they take so many years to grow or cause any symptoms. Just keeping an eye on them, called 'watchful waiting', is usually all that is needed. Yet some will consider treatment such as radiotherapy with its risk of side-effects.

Scans will often reveal unexpected findings. An older person may have been feeling reasonably well until they read their scan report which reveals all that has been found. My advice would be not to ask to see the report!

Incidentaloma

Incidentaloma is the medical term for tumours or cysts which have been found 'incidentally', and are not causing any symptoms and are unlikely ever to do so. They are found because a scan focused on one part of the body, and trying to answer one specific question will stumble upon other abnormalities nearby. Some of the most common findings include thyroid nodules, nodules in the lungs in non-smokers, adrenal tumours and enlarged lymph glands.[63] In an older person there is at least a fifty percent chance of finding an 'incidentaloma' in the chest and abdomen. Depending on how such results are interpreted and communicated, it can cause considerable anxiety to everyone at these unexpected findings. There is then a danger that this incidental finding leads to diagnosing something that isn't really a threat – we call this overdiagnosis. The temptation is to plan further investigations and treatments, just on the slim chance that the unexpected finding is in fact potentially serious.

Protocols are triggered following scans, particularly in relation to suspected cancer. In the attempt to improve the UK's cancer success rate and diagnose cancer earlier, there are policies and procedures to ensure prompt referral of suspected cancer cases to what is known as a cancer multidisciplinary team (MDT). Hence, I might have a patient admitted after a fall, and their body scan reveals an unsuspected lump in the pancreas, thought to be an early pancreatic cancer. The person's details are referred to the regional centre, where the scans will be reviewed. There is no possibility that any treatment will be proposed – the cancer is causing no symptoms and an operation would be traumatic for someone living with frailty. This MDT will never meet my patient or discuss the situation with them. But there is a risk that all of this will both heighten worries for my patient and their family, and lengthen the stay in hospital while the case is being reviewed.

Choosing wisely

There are national and international movements now seeking to highlight some of these issues under the banners of 'Too Much Medicine' and 'Choosing Wisely'. The organisation in the UK[64] describes its work like this:

Choosing Wisely UK is part of a global initiative aimed at improving conversations between patients and their doctors and nurses. By having discussions that are informed by the doctor but take into account what's important to the patient too, both sides can be supported to make better decisions

---

[63] O'Sullivan JW *et al* (2018); 'Prevalence and outcomes of incidental imaging findings: umbrella review'; BMJ 2018;361:k2387

[64] www.choosingwisely.co.uk/about-choosing-wisely-uk

about care. Often, this will help to avoid tests, treatments or procedures that are unlikely to be of benefit. Across the UK, there is a growing culture of overuse of medical intervention, with variation in the use of certain treatments across the country.

Choosing Wisely recommends four questions to be asked when an investigation or treatment is proposed, and these are highly relevant to the context of decision-making with reference to someone who is older with frailty:

1. What are the potential benefits?
2. What are the risks?
3. What are the alternatives?
4. What if I do nothing?

By asking these questions with those living with frailty, we may realise that a light touch is best. Older people grew up before the advent of the NHS and certainly before the development of modern healthcare. They are often of the view that doctors know best and may prefer to hand over decision-making. Yet this places them at risk of over-investigation, over-diagnosis and over-treatment, if doctors follow the usual pathways. These four questions can be used to assist patient-centred communication and are a great structure for the conversation with the doctor.

Traditionally doctors on qualifying swore the Hippocratic Oath, originating from 460 BC. This required doctors to commit to *primum non nocere* – "first do no harm". A retired neurosurgeon, Henry Marsh, in his book with this title[65], reflected on the difficult decisions in his specialty and the risks of being overzealous as it is so hard to do nothing. In truth there is always something doctors can do, but perhaps the starting point for treating those nearing the end of their lives should be "first do no harm".

It is too simplistic to claim ageism when looking at statistics showing lower rates of treatment for those in extreme old age. For each disease or situation, it is more complex, quite apart from individual choice and preference. Heart valve surgery illustrates the progress with modern medicine and the difficult decisions thrown up as a result. The aortic valve commonly furs up as we age, and this can cause angina and

---

[65] Marsh, Henry (2014); *Do No Harm;* Orion Books

breathlessness. For some there can be little warning until suddenly the heart gives up completely. Surgery to replace the valve is much safer today and improves symptoms. For those living with frailty, helping symptoms is probably appreciated more than extending life. A recent study[66] found that half of the subjects with moderate frailty reported some improvement in breathlessness after surgery to replace the valve, but quality of life was judged much the same, or worse, a year later. This is because so many factors influence wellbeing in those with frailty. And one quarter of those with frailty had died within a year. Knowing the right thing to do is hard, but requires good listening and a strong dose of humility.

Another good illustration of the importance of shared decision-making is when deciding whether to start kidney dialysis. Improvements in dialysis have meant that those with extreme old age and frailty are by no means excluded from dialysis. Letting the doctor decide for us can lead to starting dialysis and then regretting the decision a few months later. Dialysis is demanding in terms of days spent in the hospital for treatment and does not restore well-being as much as may be hoped. It can prolong life for some but not all; some will survive without dialysis for a long time even with very poor kidney function, enabling a 'middle way' with supportive treatments but avoiding the demands of dialysis.

In the US, expenditure on healthcare is around double that in the UK, and yet life expectancy and health is no better on average than in the UK. Dr Muriel Gillick, in her book *The Denial of Ageing*[67], describes life for many older people in Florida:

> *The average elderly Floridian sees multiple specialists, often making more than one physician visit each week. Gathered round the table, they exchange doctor stories. When one member of the group reports they have seen a new specialist, the others eagerly add the new doctor to their own lists of providers. ... What its citizens get in exchange for this largesse*

---

[66] Goudzwaard JA *et al* (2020); 'Impact of frailty on health-related quality of life 1 year after transcatheter aortic valve implantation'; Age Ageing 49:989-994

[67] THE DENIAL OF AGEING: PERPETUAL YOUTH, ETERNAL LIFE, AND OTHER DANGEROUS FANTASIES by Muriel R. Gillick, M.D., Cambridge, Mass.: Harvard University Press, Copyright © 2006 by the President and Fellows of Harvard College.

is more hospital days, more tests, more ICU admissions, and more subspeciality consultations in the last 6 months of life, with no evidence that the additional attention improves the quality of care.

In my experience, older people were enormously grateful for the treatments they received. However, they would be the first to say they would prefer the money spent on someone younger. I must have heard it said to me hundreds of times: "Why are you bothering about me? I've had my life," or words to that effect. We should allow our elderly relatives to refuse treatments if this is through a combination of not wishing to face the upheaval themselves combined with altruism towards others.

Where is the truth found?

Using the word 'truth' will make Christians think about Jesus – "I am the way, the truth, and the life."[68] In the context of healthcare, it makes us want to be assured of honesty and being told the truth by our doctors. Yet what we have discussed in this chapter shows how it is not so straightforward, especially with ageing bodies where nothing is quite perfect or certain any longer. Healthcare runs the risk of seeing us as a machine – and tests identify where the machine is not working. We can do this with amazing detail today. Yet we are made in the image of God, and the truth about us is so much more unique and mysterious. It may be that multiple parts can't be fixed, but what matters most to us? The compassionate truth is perhaps found less in the test result than in the trust rooted in the doctor-patient relationship. In my clinic at the hospital, I would sometimes pick up from the body language of the patient, or perhaps their relative, that I was perhaps not being told the whole truth. That had to wait to be revealed by the relative to the clinic nurse in a quiet moment and passed on to me subsequently.

John's Gospel says some interesting things about truth. He uses the word fifty times. John sees truth not so much as a theological treatise, but as about encountering the person of Jesus. For Jews, finding the true way to live had been about following hundreds of rules, some of which would contravene each other. Jesus condensed the rules to two over-arching commandments: to love God; and to love our neighbour as

---

[68] John 14:6 (NIV)

ourselves. All about relationships. He would most perceptively speak truth into people's lives – for the woman at the well about her sexual partners; for the rich man about being wedded to his possessions; for the paralysed man by the pool about whether he really wanted to let go of his sick role; for the pharisee Nicodemus about allowing the Holy Spirit into his dutiful life. For all these people, and many others through Gospel stories, Jesus speaks truth into their life and brings the offer of freedom. To those who put their trust in Jesus, he says, "Then you will know the truth, and the truth will set you free."[69] Jesus also showed that there are times and situations when the rules of the Sabbath must be set aside in favour of compassion:

> *On a Sabbath Jesus was teaching in one of the synagogues, and a woman was there who had been crippled by a spirit for eighteen years. She was bent over and could not straighten up at all. When Jesus saw her, he called her forward and said to her, 'Woman, you are set free from your infirmity.'[70]*

This could provide an interesting perspective on the proper place of guidelines and tests in healthcare. Understanding and strengthening the relationship between doctor and patient can point to the truth sometimes better than a whole set of tests. GPs have an advantage here over hospital doctors because the encounter with a patient can build upon both their knowledge of that person and the trust established over the years. Some would say this is more difficult today than in the past, with more part-time doctors and less emphasis on seeing 'your own doctor'. Guidelines and pathways have a very important part to play in driving up standards of healthcare and reducing the risk of mistakes. But pathways are not always compassionate. They are the product of our amazing medical science and inherently dispassionate. The trust we as doctors place in this medical knowledge can make us arrogant in thinking we know best. We are inclined to believe that the truth always lies in the scan result. But in healthcare for those living with frailty should humility play a larger part?

Humility is not always to be found in the headlines of healthcare – exaggerated and overoptimistic claims are far more common, as in the latest procedure that claims to halve deaths from cancer, or the latest pill

---

[69] John 8:32 (NIV)
[70] Luke 13:12 (NIV)

that might prevent a hundred thousand strokes. Doctors can insist on doing more tests, even when they are not sure this will lead to any change in the treatment that can be given. Likewise, families can be demanding and pressurise doctors into further tests just to be sure nothing is missed.

In caring for those living with frailty, I have tried to learn the humility of accepting the limitations of medicine and living within uncertainty. We all need to understand this and not be too demanding. Where care is more likely than cure much of the time, the truth will be found in honesty, compassion and kindness in the doctor-patient partnership. There is healing to be found in a smile, a touch, an embrace and a listening ear. The Bishop of Gloucester, Rachel Treweek, has described this beautifully: "I have personally discovered that human wholeness requires endless touches of loving restoration as we live in relationship with God and neighbour."[71] How urgently we need to re-establish the ministry of touch as we emerge from COVID. Those of us working in healthcare are fortunate to be supported by the prayers of so many – I am often embarrassed by this, feeling that everyone is equally in need of intercessory prayer. Yet I do believe that any consistency in tenderness and love I was able to show to my patients was only possible through the transforming power of God's Spirit working in my life.

So what can I make of all this?

There is no need today for older people to say, "It's just my age" – we should seek advice when there are problems, as healthcare can always help in some way. But not all tests are essential – some tests seek to rule out a diagnosis which was never very likely, and others have little chance of changing the treatment planned – yet every test can be demanding to undergo and sometimes even risky. The growth of our technological medicine, combined with the search for certainty in a climate of risk aversion, all combine to increase the number of tests that are carried out. For all of us, but especially for those living with frailty, it is important to remember that we can refuse further tests without upsetting our doctor or breaking our relationship with them. The four questions described earlier can help us decide whether to agree to a test or treatment, making sure the doctors understand a little about who we are and what matters

---

[71] Rachel Treweek (2020); *Encounters – Jesus, Connection and Story; Past, Present and Future;* Darton, Longman and Todd; p.84

most to us. As Christians, ultimately we place our trust in God, as we ask God to bring His healing in His way and in His time.

For you to consider

- Do I tend not to trouble the doctor and not ask for help when I should?
- Do I tend to worry it might be more serious and ask for more tests?
- Have I memorised the four questions to use when considering a new treatment or operation?
- Can I put my trust in God's hands for the future?

CHAPTER FIVE

Trolley Waits

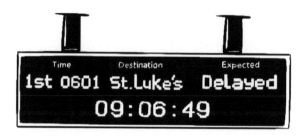

Finally, all of you, be like-minded, be sympathetic, love one another, be compassionate and humble.[72]

I WONDER WHAT YOUR LAST EXPERIENCE OF GOING INTO hospital in an emergency was like as an older person, or perhaps accompanying an older person into the NHS? The headlines are not encouraging: "Record number of A&E 'trolley waits' reached in January, NHS say" (*Guardian*, February 2020). The picture painted by the TV dramas such as *Casualty* is where staff have time to discuss their personal lives and every patient brought in seems to have a cubicle waiting for them. *24 Hours in A/E* records live action but is still more likely to focus on the dramatic or serious rather than the mundane. Older people come to hospital with the whole spectrum of illness and injury, some desperately ill, while others will come for reassurance that nothing serious is amiss. But regardless of the seriousness of the problem, the truth is that a visit to hospital can be a daunting and often harrowing experience for most older people, especially those living with frailty. There is widespread knowledge of the delays in being seen and treated in the emergency department (ED), yet this does not seem to stem the tide of demand.

---

[72] 1 Peter 3:8 (NIV)

A typical experience?

So, was your recent experience in ED anything like Amanda's?

Amanda had a telephone call from her mother Pat one morning, saying she felt very unwell and had phoned the GP. Pat was eighty-six and housebound because of her arthritis, so her walking was limited. She just managed to get round downstairs with a walking frame. She also had to keep an eye on her husband David who, although suffering from dementia, was more able physically than herself. Amanda lived two hours away and decided to cancel plans and drive over in the afternoon. Pat's GP phoned at lunchtime, not knowing Pat well, and was unsure what was causing the problem. He suspected she needed a more thorough assessment at the hospital. A paramedic arrived at the end of the afternoon and delivered Pat to the hospital on a busy evening. She was taken into 'majors' and helped on to a trolley in the corridor, waiting to see someone. There was so much noise and bustle – nurses and doctors passing by – but no-one came to see them. It was difficult for either of them to relax. Pat's first assessment was with a nurse, and she was told she would see the doctor later. Pat was now desperate for the toilet and Amanda felt somewhat helpless. Finally, she managed to catch a nurse who kindly brought a commode. A doctor tried to take a history, but Pat had forgotten to bring her hearing aid, so Amanda provided what details she knew.

By 9pm Pat had had blood tests and an X-ray, but she now needed to be seen by the on-call medical team. Amanda heard them muttering something about a urine infection. Pat was getting more anxious about David on his own at home and really just wanted to go home. To help calm Pat, Amanda decided to go back to the house to check on David. Pat moved off the corridors and onto a bed on the medical ward at 3am, and went through the story again with one of the medical team as best she could. Next morning, she was seen by the duty consultant who explained that she had some constipation and a possible urinary infection and could go home. Amanda tried to phone the ward twice but got no reply. Pat had hardly moved off the bed, having been on a trolley yesterday for ten hours, without her usual painkillers, and felt very stiff. The physiotherapist came and gave her a new frame but decided she would not manage to get into a car to go home. The ward phoned Amanda at home, who was relieved finally to hear the plan and reassured the ward she would stay with David. The hospital transport arrived to collect her at 5.30pm. Unbelievably, her new pills were left at the hospital – but amazingly, an apologetic hospital nurse offered to drop them off on her way home that night.

But imagine that story without Amanda there to help... The anxiety would have been worse, and who knows what could have happened to David overnight? During this relatively short time in hospital there are so many things that can go wrong. Pat could have been incontinent and that could have caused skin problems. She could easily have got stuck on the trolley and been unable to walk the next morning, necessitating even longer in hospital. She could have fallen off the trolley and sustained a serious injury. She could have become confused with the many moves and disrupted routine and a long day. Her husband could have wandered out of the house in the late evening trying to find her. And so on. She was shown kindness throughout, but was it all necessary?

Another fall

For those living with frailty, around a quarter of attendances at the emergency department are after a fall. Their fragility means that nasty injuries occur even just from slipping to the floor in the house. First Aid is often insufficient to deal with complex skin wounds, while bones are broken so easily. The trauma units know that hidden internal damage and bleeding can be substantial, so whole-body scans as well as X-rays are required to reveal the full picture. These scans can create some difficult decisions for treatment as illustrated by Mildred.

Mildred was a lady of ninety-two years. She lived in a large modern nursing home in our city and had been there for three years with her worsening Alzheimer's disease. She got on well with the staff but had almost forgotten her family who lived an hour away. She fell one night in her room; she was a frequent faller and was probably trying to get to the toilet, forgetting she was unable to walk. She took no regular medication now; I had stopped them all on her last visit to the hospital – pills she previously took to lower blood pressure and prevent stroke – because they also increased her risk of falling. Staff at the home felt she was her usual self but noted a small bruise on her head and did not wish to be blamed for any negligence. So, the nurse on duty had phoned the paramedics who could not be sure there was no brain damage from the head injury and referred her to the hospital. This meant an ambulance journey at night and lying on a hospital trolley in the emergency department.

The doctor in the ED assessing Mildred referred her for a CT scan of her head and neck to look for any serious injury. The scan revealed a small subdural haemorrhage – a bruise on the surface of the brain – and also a broken bone in her neck called the odontoid peg. The guidelines for these conditions meant her brain scan was discussed with the regional neurosurgeons, and the neck fracture with the local orthopaedic surgeons. The neurosurgeon advised admission for forty-eight hours' observation, while the orthopaedic advice was to wear a neck brace for eight weeks. I met Mildred the next morning on a trolley in the corridor. She was agitated, confused and distressed, and frequently fiddling with her uncomfortable neck brace. I knew from numerous conversations with the neurosurgeons for similar cases that they would be very reluctant to operate and would prefer to let the haemorrhage resolve on its own. I could also see that a neck brace for eight weeks would be very distressing, and probably impractical. I knew she would be more settled back at her nursing home, where the staff would be best able to observe any changes in her condition. She stayed with us for twenty-four hours to be sure the neck fracture was not causing any nerve damage or pain. The nurse in charge at the home was only too pleased to have Mildred back without the brace. I also had a lovely chat with her son on the telephone, who just wanted Mum to be looked after in the home. She actually had a RESPECT form (see chapter eight) which stated "to be treated at home if possible" – more precise wording might have avoided hospital attendance altogether.

Mildred was a complex case: the evidence around the right thing to do for an odontoid fracture is controversial. This fracture occurs very easily in old people, but thankfully rarely causes nerve damage. The brace allows time for the bones to knit together – but in around eighty percent the bones never heal. The brace is very uncomfortable and, especially for someone with severe dementia, hard to tolerate, and risks poor swallowing and increased confusion. Likewise, the usual management plan for a subdural haemorrhage is to observe in hospital and repeat the scan a few days later – but the staff at the care home could provide much better supervision knowing Mildred, and further scans to show whether the haemorrhage was increasing would still be unlikely to lead to surgery. The case illustrates the dilemma thrown up by scans, and compassionate, pragmatic decision-making rather than the usual pathway – the 'middle way' we explored in chapter four.

Kept in overnight

For someone over seventy-five without frailty, the chance of an admission to hospital in any year is around one in ten; for those living with severe frailty it reaches nine out of ten. People over the age of seventy-five are over-represented in ED; they account for seventeen percent of ED attendances in England, although they make up only eight percent of the population. Around two thirds of these attendances become a hospital admission – over the age of eighty-five it is over three quarters. This contrasts to only a fifth of younger people being admitted. We might think this difference is because older people coming to hospital are much more ill. But actually the difference in admission rate has a lot to do with practicalities:

- *Communication*
  Is there someone able to give a good history of what has happened?
- *Support*
  Is there someone able to help the person when they get back home?
- *Transport*
  Is there some means of transporting back home?

If someone is being admitted to hospital from the ED, they need to wait for a bed to become available. That is usually where the problem starts. Hospitals are full all the time – a bed becomes available only because another person has just been discharged. The number of NHS hospital bed numbers has halved over the last thirty years,[73] while the aged population has been increasing. The only way this works is by steadily reducing the length of stay in hospital. But while waiting for a bed to become available, the person will be placed on a trolley and, in most hospitals, will stay in the ED or in a corridor very nearby. And they may then be on a trolley for a long time; in January 2020 there were 2,846 'trolley waits' longer than twelve hours, compared to 647 twelve-

---

[73] Kings Fund (2020); 'NHS hospital bed numbers'

hour waits in January 2019.[74] And given that older people are commonly the ones being admitted, they are disproportionately the ones lying on those trolleys for hours. Not surprisingly, there are occasions when someone will die in the corridor while they are waiting for a space on the ward. This does not necessarily mean that their life could have been saved, as treatments such as drips or antibiotics may well have been administered already. But clearly it is a terrible experience, devoid of dignity and compassion.

Compassion under stress

If you have accompanied someone into a busy ED, I am sure you will be able to echo a number of those experiences and add some of your own. No doubt you were also grateful for the attention and care given amidst all the stress and worry.

There are moments of stress in Jesus' ministry captured in the Gospel narratives. For example, Mark describes how Jesus was preaching to crowds by the lakeside having just returned from healing a demon-possessed man. He responds to a desperate request to visit Jairus' daughter who is dying, and starts on the journey surrounded by crowds following Him. In the midst of all this, He is aware of a woman touching His cloak and healing power going out to her. He stops and they converse. And then a further message comes through from Jairus' home that his daughter has died. But Jesus says to Jairus, "Don't be afraid. Just have faith and she will be healed."[75] The calm in Jesus' words and actions contrasts starkly with all the pressure around and is a shining example for those of us who work in busy hospitals. That too is a reminder for us to pray for all the staff who feel hard-pressed, not knowing which way to turn as so many are needing attention.

Three Gospel writers describe this story, but only Mark details the woman's dealings with the medical profession of the day: "She had suffered a great deal from many doctors, and over the years she had spent everything she had to pay them, but she had got no better."[76] This is not mentioned by Luke, the physician! Jesus' compassion for all those He meets who are suffering is described in the strongest possible way. We

---

[74] *Daily Mail,* 13th Feb 2020; 'Twelve-hour A&E wait times quadruple in a single year, the worst on record'; dailymail.co.uk

[75] Luke 8:50 (NLT)

[76] Mark 5:26 (NLT)

may use the word 'pity', but this can sound patronising and therefore dispassionate. The Greek word used in the Gospels is *splanchnizomai,* which literally means 'being moved in your guts' – gut-wrenching compassion. For Jesus, compassion always wins over the rules. But my concern, and indeed my observation over the years, is that in healthcare, the guidelines and pathways can easily dominate and trump compassion. The closely balanced margins of benefits over risks from medical interventions in older people living with frailty are not understood sufficiently by healthcare staff or, if they are understood, not sufficiently explained to patients. Sometimes the courageous and compassionate decision is *not* to follow the guidelines, to avoid the danger of over-medicalising. And this can mirror the experience of this woman with bleeding.

The healing of the woman from what we presume was menorrhagia – persistent heavy periods – is a story of restored dignity as well as physical healing. The woman was able to take her place again in society, to meet others and attend temple worship. Jesus loves to restore dignity to the outcast, as He meets people who have been disabled for many years, analogous to the chronic conditions we see in old age today. He heals a woman who has been crippled and bent over for eighteen years, perhaps with severe osteoporosis, who is released "from her bondage". Two blind beggars cry out for mercy, and having received their sight back, they begin a new life and follow Jesus. Meeting a man with leprosy, Jesus, "moved with compassion, reached out and touched him"[77] and in so doing restored the man's identity and dignity, enabling him to live with others again. All of these examples show Jesus restoring dignity as part of the healing. How can the hospital show this dignity and compassion to the most fragile, while seeking to provide healing?

The challenge to change

Countless reports have acknowledged that our current models of care must change to reflect the growing proportion of patients presenting with complex needs related to frailty. The principles of how to care for older people are widely taught, and yet hospitals still struggle to deliver an age-friendly service. Hospitals up and down the land have acknowledged the need for change and are embarrassed when reports of appalling standards of care emerge. There were campaigns such as The British Geriatrics

---

[77] Mark 1:41 (NLT)

Society's 'Behind Closed Doors'[78] in 2006 to improve privacy and dignity, especially around toileting, and the creation of 'dignity champions' in 2006. And then in 2009 some horrific standards of care were revealed at the Mid Staffs Hospitals Trust which led to the Francis Inquiry and the Berwick report on patient safety.

How great are the risks in hospital for someone with frailty?

Much of the problem for those with frailty is balancing the necessity to receive urgent or necessary treatment with the almost unavoidable risks of being in hospital. Let me explain some of the principal risks which continue today.

- One of the highest risks for anyone staying in hospital is *acquiring another infection*. This is termed 'healthcare associated infection'. Overall about eight percent of admissions are complicated by an infection, but this is higher for those living with frailty. The consequence can be serious: a longer stay or even proving fatal. Infections that have acquired notoriety are norovirus and *Clostridium difficile* which both cause diarrhoea, and MRSA which can cause wound infections. But a whole range of organisms cause infections in the skin, chest and urine as well. The likelihood of infection is influenced by how many tubes or drips are present, along with age and frailty. Unfortunately, the immune system is much weaker in those with frailty. To make matters worse, the infections picked up in hospital are often more resistant to antibiotics, and so more difficult to cure, than infections at home.
- *Falls in hospital* are also common for someone living with frailty. With a ten-day admission, the risk of a fall is about one in eight. While many of those falls will result in nothing worse than some bruising, some will result in a fracture such as a broken hip. Having a fall will often add another week to the hospital stay, and greatly upset confidence.
- *Becoming confused* while in hospital is very common, especially for those who already have some memory loss. This is called delirium, and can extend the time in hospital, as well as permanently damage the brain. It occurs in around one in four

---

[78] British Geriatrics Society; Behind Closed Doors Tools.pdf; bgs.org.uk

admissions for an older person with frailty. There are many causes for delirium: it can be due to the illness, or just the huge interruption of routines and lack of familiarity of everything around them. There is no effective treatment for delirium, but we do know some things which help to avoid it, such as maintaining good sight and hearing, minimising some medication, keeping up with eating and drinking, and being in touch with familiar people such as their family.

- *Losing strength and becoming weaker* occurs surprisingly quickly, and if someone only has enough strength to walk or get out of a chair on their own, then the loss of strength following being in bed for a few days can make a crucial difference. Some studies indicate we can lose ten to fifteen percent of our muscle strength from just ten days in bed, and this seems to be faster in older people than the young. Yet remaining in bed seems to be part of the 'hospital experience' for most.

- Weakness is accelerated by *poor nutrition,* and this is another challenge in hospital, affecting up to half of older people. The reasons are multiple and include: a reduced appetite when ill; not having the food that someone has been used to for many years, or at the wrong time; trying to eat while lying in bed.

- *Losing an independent spirit and becoming depressed* is called institutionalisation. Life at home for someone with frailty is often a struggle, but the daily routines are sustaining. Lose those routines and things seem to fall apart quite quickly.

It is all quite sobering. For those living with significant frailty, personhood is so easily diminished by a spell in hospital; indeed, one of the pleasures in geriatric medicine is meeting your patient again after a hospital admission, in the clinic, in their home or in the street, and seeing their personhood restored – perhaps understanding for the first time who they really are.

The benefits of the admission are likely to be greatest in the first few days, while the risks increase steadily the longer the admission. Even the best care in hospital will only reduce the risk of these adverse events a little.

So what does an age-friendly hospital look like?

Some of the most important ingredients for an age-friendly hospital might seem to have little to do with the medical care. There is the need to cater for poor mobility, with the availability of walking aids if they were not brought in the ambulance, and easy access to disabled toilets nearby. There need to be plentiful chairs, as it is safer to sit on an armchair rather than lie on a hospital bed or trolley whenever possible. Communication aids may help the deaf who do not have a hearing aid, and clear signs and directions may help them avoid going round in circles. A trolley service for snacks and drinks is much appreciated. For those living with frailty, these things can make an enormous difference to a good outcome at the end of the day. Everyone knows these things are important. Feedback to a ward or department can be given, for example by using the 'friends and family' cards, and this will help to improve standards. These standards are also assessed by the Care Quality Commission in their regular inspections of hospitals. The latest report for each hospital is published on the internet for anyone to read.

VISITORS ARE CRUCIAL

Visits from family and carers can be vital for older people, and especially for those living with dementia or frailty. In the past, hospitals often restricted visiting hours, as visitors can be seen to hamper hospital routines and be over-demanding of staff time. The curtailment of hospital visiting during the COVID crisis has been another tragic aspect of the pandemic. John's Campaign[79] was started by a family in 2017 to encourage hospitals to offer open visiting hours for patients with dementia, and to make a bed available overnight for a carer if needed.

John was in hospital for five weeks with a leg ulcer and subsequent norovirus. John went in strong, mobile, smiling, able to tell stories about his past, work in his garden and help with things round the house. He was able to feed himself, to keep clean, to have a good kind of daily life. He came out skeletal, immobile, incoherent, requiring twenty-four-hour care and barely knowing those around him. His family are sure that if he had not spent that time alone without them, he would not have descended into such a state of deep delirium.

---

[79] johnscampaign.org.uk

Having someone with us – someone whom we love, whom we know, whose face we know (be they our carer, our family, our friend, our lover) – helps keep us tied to reality, to life, to sanity.

Most hospitals in the UK have now signed up to John's Campaign.

LAST 1000 DAYS

There has been another campaign in recent years called *#Last1000days*, which emphasises the importance of time when you don't have much time left. For those living with frailty, time is precious. Just as no-one looks back on their life and says, "I wish I had spent longer in the office," it is unlikely that anyone wishes they had spent longer in the hospital! Pat and Amanda's story at the start of this chapter was probably not a waste of time, yet could have been managed quicker. But do we need a radically different and special approach for our frail elders?

FRAILTY TEAMS

The time spent in the whole process is one of the most stressful elements of the experience. Many EDs now have a 'frailty team' working there, although perhaps only during the day, who can short-circuit the process described above and bring the consultant decision much earlier. This can increase the number of people able to be discharged home the same day. I myself developed such a service in my hospital which grew to assessing over twenty people each day, half of whom would be able to go home the same day, a marked improvement on the 'usual service' where up to eighty percent would stay in for at least a night. We spot vulnerable older people as soon after their arrival as possible and see if we can work with them and their family to find quick solutions to their problems. Our frailty team consists of consultants and registrars who have specialised in the care of older people, working with advanced nurse practitioners – experienced and trained in holistic care of the needs of older people. The team undertakes assessments in a separate area in the ED, and later on the admissions ward. The noise and bustle in an ED are upsetting for older people, and a quieter, more peaceful environment helps everyone. In the assessment unit the team is supported by therapists, a pharmacist for a medication review and discharge coordinators. The latter are amazing 'fixers' who manage to short-circuit bureaucracy and arrange appropriate support to enable a same day or next day discharge. Different versions of this team are appearing right across the UK and are starting to transform the experience for those with frailty presenting to the hospital.

Hospital-at-home

What if the acute illness was able to be managed without coming to hospital at all? GPs manage hundreds of less severe problems without hospital treatment, but for those living with frailty, the diagnosis underlying the problem can often be far from obvious and may need some simple tests to sort out. In most parts of the country a service referred to as hospital-at-home, sometimes known as 'rapid response', brings a team specialising in the care of older people and frailty out to the house, and they will have access to tests and medical support. Local surveys almost always show this service is very highly regarded by those who have been treated by them – patients will say, "Please, can I have that team again if ever I need urgent help!"

One example of a condition that can often be managed at home with less need for admission to hospital is heart failure. Heart failure is a long term condition which has become more common these days; thanks to very successful treatment of heart attacks, more people will survive the initial attack, but as a consequence some will be left with a weakened heart, termed 'heart failure'. The condition has been greatly improved by a number of medications, which both help symptoms and prolong survival. The condition can flare up at any time, and this can lead to an emergency admission. But the hospital-at-home team can give all the treatment for this at home very successfully.

The hospital-at-home teams also treat pneumonia at home with oxygen and injected antibiotics if needed.[80] This is a wonderful way of still giving active treatment yet respecting the person's wish to remain at home. This has been used extensively throughout the COVID crisis. And research has shown that older people being treated at home for pneumonia fare just as well as those going into hospital, but with a better quality of life experience. The teams can support many conditions, such as a minor stroke or the consequences of a fall. Important tests such as an X-ray or scan can be arranged urgently by liaison with the hospital-based frailty team. Brian illustrated a typical pathway.

---

[80] Caplan GA (1999); 'Hospital in the home: a randomised clinical trial'; Med J Aust1999 Feb 15;170(4):156-60

I met Brian one late morning on a trolley in the emergency department. He had been sent up urgently by his GP as he had become more breathless through the night. Brian knew he had heart failure and took all his pills religiously. He had noticed over the last week that his legs were swelling up again, and then the breathlessness worsened, although he had not done anything out of the ordinary. He didn't want to come into hospital but knew he needed help. My assessment in ED confirmed the diagnosis of heart failure, but his blood tests also showed he had a longstanding degree of kidney failure. The letter from the GP indicated that the kidney failure was the reason his diuretics had not been increased. Thankfully, his oxygen level was only marginally below what it should be. Our team administered a diuretic injection and I adjusted his medication. We phoned the hospital-at-home team and asked them to treat him at home. They arranged oxygen which would be at the house later that day. They would visit at the end of the day to give another injection if needed and would visit three or four times a day over the next few days. This all went to plan – Brian was feeling much better after our initial treatment in hospital. The hospital-at-home nurse phoned me the next day to give a report on his progress and discuss the result of that day's blood test. Brian was delighted when I met him for review in the clinic the following week!

Some people have their condition monitored with simple equipment at home as well. This sort of management is called telehealth, and can help people with chronic lung conditions, reducing the need for emergency admissions. Both GPs and hospital doctors can refer people to these telehealth services, which are completely free. Specialist nurses attached to the telehealth service teach how to monitor the condition and how to spot the earliest signs of things going awry. They give advice either if the person is concerned or if the monitoring has shown a change in measurements which may need new or adjusted medication.

Older people are special

Modern healthcare systems are designed around efficiency and technical expertise, and centralisation of services has been necessary to deliver this. But how does this fit with the preferences of those living with frailty, those who are most vulnerable to risk? The system is designed around reducing the risk of missing a serious diagnosis, yet for those with frailty there may be fewer options for intervention – at least without substantially increasing the risk of damaging complications from a longer spell in hospital. The American geriatrician Muriel Gillick[81] put it like this in 2006:

> *The more radical approach would be to avoid hospitalisation altogether. Rather than proceed with "usual care" while trying to minimise its deleterious consequences, why not simply avoid "usual care". If hospitals are too toxic to older people, why not try to treat them at home rather than administer antitoxins?*

There is arrogance in a system that believes there is only one correct way to manage an illness. Frailty medicine – the style of medicine practiced by hospital-at-home teams and frailty units – has developed a person-centred middle way; it is neither the 'usual' way nor one of palliation and 'just keep comfortable'. This middle way – with a light touch – is comfortable with uncertainty. We saw in the previous chapter that certainty is elusive, and pursuit of certainty only leads to more tests.

An illustration of finding a middle way is around infection and possible sepsis. Infection becomes sepsis when the body is making an excessive immune response which is actually harmful. 'Sepsis 6' is a protocol to signal possible sepsis, with a set of actions which can save many lives. Septic shock will usually require management in an intensive care unit and has a high fatality rate in the very old. But for those with frailty, some of those sepsis signs are present even without infection and are not such a reliable indicator of impending septic shock. A large majority of infections never become sepsis. The protocol necessitates admission to hospital, with repeated blood tests and monitoring of urine by a catheter. This is often linked to the protocol around acute kidney injury, which is also promoted to save lives. Kidney function is commonly a little worse during any illness for those living with frailty. These protocols have a momentum of their own, which pushes aside any other considerations, such as patient preference. The middle way makes pragmatic decisions for those with frailty, and perhaps fewer tests, with

---

[81] THE DENIAL OF AGEING: PERPETUAL YOUTH, ETERNAL LIFE, AND OTHER DANGEROUS FANTASIES by Muriel R. Gillick, M.D., Cambridge, Mass.: Harvard University Press, Copyright © 2006 by the President and Fellows of Harvard College.

treatment that gives a reasonable chance of success, within the constraints of uncertainty – this is often termed empirical treatment.

Not everyone will choose this alternative way – some will wish to accept the risks of hospitalisation in pursuit of hi-tech treatment. The substantial growth of emergency community services such as hospital-at-home, and frailty units in our hospitals, is creating this special service for those living with frailty, but more innovation is needed to refine and develop these approaches. I believe this middle way can show respect and honour to our older people and may reflect the compassion of Jesus.

St Paul wrote, "...those parts of the body that seem to be weaker are indispensable, and the parts that we think are less honourable we treat with special honour."[82] Respecting older people living with frailty requires us to respect their choices and preferences, even if at times we do not agree. This might be one of the steps in letting go.

Healing in frailty

As Christians we believe in God's power to heal today, which God does partly through the hands of those working in the health services, and partly through the human body's own wonderful capacity to heal and recover itself, all aided by faithful prayers. I believe God enables miraculous cures, sometimes through prayer ministry, and the Holy Spirit can prompt us in how to pray for those we love. As a consultant there were numerous times where recovery against all the odds surprised me. We have discussed facing the reality of ageing in chapter two, and by 'healing' we cannot mean curing the ageing process. Curing means eradicating the disease, whereas healing is all about making whole again. For the diseases of old age and frailty, most cannot be cured. But healing is possible without cure: making sense and coming to terms with our condition; improving the symptoms so that we can live with it; and even using it for a new purpose – these are all possibilities when we are 'healed'. Healing restores our equilibrium. And as Christians that means we are free again to live for God.

Muriel was an eighty-five-year-old widow I met one day. She had been unwell in a vague way for several months, not eating, and feeling cross with herself that she was so tired. She had some blood test results which worried her GP, who referred her urgently to my care. I

---

[82] 1 Corinthians 12:22-23 (NIV)

arranged a liver scan, and this sadly showed up a probable cancer. I had to explain to her the findings, and that given her age and the position of the cancer, there was no treatment that could be offered. I listened to her concerns. She held my hand, looked straight at me and said she was so glad to know that there was something behind it all. She was so grateful for the clear explanation and the brief kindness shown by the staff, which embarrassed us; we felt we had done so little. I gave her a pill to help improve her appetite, and arranged to see her next month. At her review, she was still smiling, and feeling better. She told me that after I had broken the news to her, she had been in contact with her estranged son and he had been to see her.

In my work I would frequently pray for wisdom to know how we might bring healing to the situation, in whatever way that might mean. Remember how Jesus said to the blind Bartimaeus, "What do you want me to do for you?"[83] We all need to pray for wisdom to know how to pray for those who are ill. When we pray for healing, it may be for physical healing, but always for wholeness.

For you to consider

- Have you an emergency plan to swing into action when a medical crisis occurs?
- Have you witnessed some of the adverse events of being in hospital with frailty?
- Are you aware of the alternatives to an emergency department or hospital admission in your area?
- Do you think the alternatives are ageist?

---

[83] Mark 10:51 (NIV)

CHAPTER SIX

When the Mind is Troubled

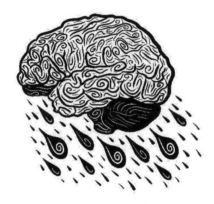

Thou wilt keep him in perfect peace, whose mind is stayed on thee: because he trusteth in thee.[84]

MY WIFE IS FAR MORE SOCIABLE THAN ME. FROM TIME TO time, she will be on the telephone chatting to a friend, and it will not be unusual at some point for the conversation to turn to parents and health concerns. As the conversation progresses, my wife might ask her friend if she would like a word with me about the situation. "Oh, I wouldn't want to trouble him." "No, it is fine; he would be happy to have a chat." The phone will be passed across, and I hear something like this:

"She is just not looking after herself – she has so many tablets, and I don't think she is taking them properly so how can she expect to be any better? I think she has been worse since the last lot of tablets. But I worry about her memory – she says some very odd things sometimes and gets muddled about our children. She got completely lost coming back from the shops this week and phoned me in a great state. But then another day we can have a laugh and a lovely conversation about the past. I don't

---

[84]   Isaiah 26:2 (KJV)

want to upset her – she insists she is fine and doesn't want any help. Do you think I should take her to the doctor? Does this sound like Alzheimer's to you?"

The stigma of mental illness

For years there has been a stigma about mental illness, and perhaps even more so for Christians. The psalmist certainly experienced a lot of depression with which we can identify, but mostly he managed to remain positive and place his trust in God to restore his spirit through an act of will: "Why are you downcast, O my soul? Why so disturbed within me? Put your hope in God, for I will yet praise Him."[85] Similarly, both Jesus and the epistle writers tell us not to be anxious, reassuring us that God, who cares for each one of us so deeply, will look after us and we need not worry about tomorrow. For some, the promises in the Bible and the support from other Christians can be enormously comforting. For others, those same promises can create a sense of false guilt as an inner voice says, "If you were a real Christian, you wouldn't be feeling this way." Admitting to depression or anxiety can look like a lack of faith.

Helping depression in frailty

Trying to put a figure on the frequency of depression for those living with frailty is probably meaningless – loss is so much a part of the experience of ageing and frailty for most people, and the spectrum of depression stretches from a sense of loneliness or reduced purpose right up to psychosis and suicide. Loss may be of friends or a lifelong partner through bereavement; or of social engagement, perhaps caused by difficulty in getting out and about. Impairment of sight or hearing compounds the sense of isolation and can add to the fear of being outside. Thankfully, persistent loneliness does not vary with age even if social contacts decrease.[86] Nevertheless, the COVID pandemic amplified loneliness and isolation, particularly for those with frailty forced into prolonged shielding and lockdown. Indeed, research has shown that anxiety, depression and loneliness doubled in older people who were shielding, even if they had maintained their telephone contacts.[87] This

---

[85] Psalm 42:5 (NIV)
[86] Age UK; 'All the lonely people; loneliness in later life'; September 2018
[87] https://www.elsa-project.ac.uk/covid-19-reports

emphasises the enormous impact of the pandemic on those living with frailty, over and above the number of deaths. Church closures were hard for an older population whose lack of IT skills made it difficult to engage with virtual church services.

For mild depression and loneliness, talking therapies and social contact are therapeutic, and the church community has an important responsibility here. Those who are struggling to engage with church should not be forgotten, and we must be ready to listen or visit. Some Psalms remain in the dark night – such as Psalms 22, 44 and 88 – and may be helpful for some who are finding it difficult to recognise God's presence; whereas in Psalms 34 and 42, for example, there is a chink of light to offer hope. Everyone has a responsibility to be aware of those living on their own and to demonstrate that God has not forgotten them. "Father of orphans and protector of widows is God in his holy habitation. God gives the desolate a home to live in."[88] Interestingly, some Bible translations of this verse say "set the lonely in families" but the meaning is probably more to emphasise the inclusiveness of God's family, the church, rather than making us feel guilty at not supporting our relatives enough. There is some evidence that severe depression is less common in regular church attenders.[89] And isolation is not inevitable when housebound – as Joy in our introduction illustrated, and for whom visitors helped sustain her faith and vitality, as well as vice versa.

Therapy options

Feelings of isolation may be helped by consistent social contact, but loneliness and depression are often more deep-seated. Unfortunately, antidepressants for most of the milder forms of late life depression have limited benefit, and talking therapies from a trained therapist or counsellor are likely to be more helpful. The antidepressants commonly bring side-effects for those with frailty – such as nausea, or increased risk of falling and confusion. Prayer and prayer ministry can bring God's healing and can definitely be therapeutic. Research has shown that Christian counselling for mild depression is just as effective or better than

---

[88] Psalm 68:5-6 (NRSV)
[89] Lawrence RE *et al* (2016); 'Religion and suicide risk'; Arch Suicide Res. 2016; 20(1): 1-21

antidepressants.[90] Therapies like Yoga and Tai Chi may be too ambitious for those with frailty, but music therapy is of proven benefit.[91] When depression is affecting the physical health of an older person with symptoms such as poor sleep, loss of appetite or loss of weight, the condition can respond well to medication. Severe forms can include delusions and paranoid thoughts – a sense of people watching or intending to do harm – which can be very upsetting for everyone. It can be difficult to distinguish severe depression from dementia, and referral to specialist mental health services is needed.

How common is dementia?

In the early stages of a dementia illness, the disease can masquerade as anxiety or depression. An antidepressant may be tried, to disentangle the altered mood from a possible dementia. Dementia also has a stigma of its own and, for those living into old age, may be feared more than cancer. Perhaps we have known someone whose life disintegrated through advanced dementia? Or known someone who was exhausted by the stress of caring for their spouse or other relative?

Dementia complicates all the issues that we are considering in this book – the risks from going into hospital, the risks of coming home and managing perhaps alone, decision-making around tests and treatments, making plans for future care, and ultimately around letting go and withdrawing treatment at the end of life. Dementia is common, and the prevalence increases rapidly as we age, almost doubling every five years: from around one in sixty at sixty-five; one in thirty at seventy; one in sixteen at seventy-five; one in ten at eighty; one in five at eighty-five; and one in three above ninety years.[92] But then let's be positive and say that two-thirds of the over nineties do not have dementia! In the UK, about two-thirds of cases are thought to have been diagnosed – the diagnosis confirmed by a GP or specialist clinic. In my experience a large proportion of those in the upper age groups have not been given a diagnosis

90 Nyer M *et al* (2013); 'What is the role of alternative treatments in late-life depression?'; Psychiatr Clin N Am 36 577-596

91 Zhao, K (2016); 'A systematic review and meta-analysis of music therapy for older adults with depression'; Geriatric Psychiatry 31:1188-1198

92 Prince, M *et al* (2014); 'Dementia UK: Update Second Edition'; report produced by King's College London and the London School of Economics for the Alzheimer's Society; p.48

– the memory problem being put down to their age, which in a sense is true. Commonly I find a relative tells me something like, "I've known for a long time that her memory is going – but she seemed to be able to pull the wool over the doctor's eyes when she went for the memory test." GPs will commonly make the diagnosis, but if they are unsure then referral to a specialist memory service will help tease out exactly what is going on. The comprehensive assessment by the doctor or community nurse (discussed in chapter three) can be a good start.

Giving it a name

June and Alastair were real stalwarts at their church, leading house-groups and prayer ministry, and Alastair, a retired teacher, was a lay reader. Perhaps the first sign of something amiss was when June, who had a beautiful reading voice, would hesitate at the lectern when reading the lesson and lose her place. Little changed for months, but Alastair increasingly realised that June's memory was failing, for example when asking an odd question while watching a TV programme or being unable to recall yesterday's conversation. June was not convinced there was a problem, but she agreed to see the GP. There she 'passed the test' and felt vindicated. Her difficulty was changing so slowly, but then an injury and hospital visits seem to bring the problem into sharper relief. June was now getting frustrated and flustered over finding the right words, while Alastair had taken over most of the domestic duties in the home. Alastair assumed the diagnosis but did not want to name it in case this alarmed her further. They contacted the local mental health team and waited months to hear anything. They wondered if anything might help.

The key pointers to a diagnosis of dementia are progressive changes over some months or years in the person's intellect, memory, and verbal and practical skills. Changes in emotions are common as well, and personality changes occur with some types of dementia. It is likely that some elements will be more noticeable than others, but some sort of combination of those changes is needed to make the diagnosis. People closest to the person are likely to be most aware of the changes, although a partner almost unconsciously makes excuses within the loving relation-ship that clouds their judgement – or perhaps they just do not want to confront the condition honestly. Sometimes it is only when the partner is out of the picture that the extent of a dementia becomes all too clear to everyone else. The suggestion of having a formal assessment can meet with anger or denial that there is anything wrong, or indeed a flat refusal to see someone; it might then be pragmatic to reach an agreement with the GP of 'presumed dementia', although this is clearly not ideal.

Blood tests follow to rule out other sometimes treatable causes for the problem such as an underactive thyroid gland. A brain scan is usually arranged for those a little younger, but in those over eighty-five or so, the scan is unlikely to change the diagnosis or management. Unfortunately, everyone's brain appears rather shrunken on a scan after that age!

The value of naming it

The value of a diagnosis is to enable some honesty about the situation, which can unlock several doors. It may lead to arranging or activating a power of attorney (see chapter eight). It may lead to a review as to whether driving is still safe. When I had these discussions in the clinic, the person typically would insist to me that they only used the car for local journeys and knew the roads very well. I might suggest a relative accompanied them on a journey, as this can provide a clear idea of whether there are problems. I would recommend a driving assessment, which can be arranged by many local authorities, or through the DVLA. I sometimes said gently to the disbelieving patient, "Why don't you just prove to your daughter that you are fine by going on a drive with an instructor?" This approach perhaps reflects Paul's advice to the younger Timothy: "Don't correct an older man. Encourage him, as you would your own father."[93] But the DVLA and insurance companies do need to be informed of a diagnosis of dementia.

The diagnosis of dementia provides a link to the local memory services for support, who can give vital training for carers in understanding dementia and how to cope with unusual behaviour. (In most parts of the country, you can refer yourself for support and advice.) At present, a diagnosis sadly does not lead to a cure, but there are treatments which can reduce the symptoms for a while. Only a half of people will respond to those drugs, and some people cannot tolerate the treatment because of side-effects. Hopefully, treatments to slow the disease will be available in the future. There are, however, other treatments which may help with symptoms such as disturbed sleeping or upsetting hallucinations. Some

---

[93] 1 Timothy 5:1 (CEV)

may find Louise Morse's publications helpful, with her Christian perspective – such as *Dementia: Frank and Linda's Story*[94].

There may come a time when care at home is exhausted and a care home seems to be the only option. Some care homes provide a day care service, and families have often told me that familiarity with a care home, either through day care or a respite admission, can ease the transition. Everyone needs a holiday break from caring, although it must also be admitted that a respite spell can be counter-productive where the person struggles in a strange environment and the carer then feels anxious or guilty. Alternatives of a family member coming to stay for a week as carer, or the person moving to another relative for a spell, are all fraught with risks – there are no perfect solutions. We think a little further about this in the next chapter.

In hospital with dementia

Dementia in old age can be thought of as frailty of the brain – it develops insidiously as reserve is lost, and might not be noticed at first. But when a crisis or stressful event occurs, from an illness or a change in circumstance, there is no brain reserve to call upon and everything falls apart. The acute confusion resulting from this is called delirium. Worried carers might contact the emergency services with their concern: she is more confused; he is not eating or drinking enough; she has gone off her feet and lost balance; he has become difficult to manage and a bit aggressive at home.

An urgent blood test is very useful in these situations, because it throws light on whether there is a medical cause underlying the delirium which requires treatment. The two most common problems revealed are dehydration and an infection. And of course, most older people with dementia have other conditions, which might be another reason for the deterioration. The dementia makes it much more difficult to obtain a clear history of what might be wrong. For all these reasons, an urgent medical assessment is important and valuable.

However, if the medical assessment and blood tests are normal, then treatment in hospital is unlikely to be helpful. Indeed, the best treatment for delirium is being cared for in one's usual home with familiar people around you and providing reassurance, while being in hospital may well

---

[94] Louise Morse (2010); *Dementia: Frank and Linda's Story;* Monarch Books

make the delirium worse. I found it was common for the tests to be normal, making it difficult to give a clear explanation for the delirium episode. This added to the stress because the carers naturally hoped that a simple cause could be found with the prospect of early treatment and resolution. With normal tests there was the likelihood of being allowed home, which might be a mixed blessing if the family were exhausted or fearful of managing any longer. This reveals the substantial gap in healthcare in most parts of the UK – the lack of urgent twenty-four-hour care and support in one's own home during an episode of delirium, perhaps because of the false assumption that the best place to be for enhanced care would be the hospital. The need for such care can be anticipated – episodes of delirium are inevitable in dementia, although obviously it is impossible to know when they might occur. So, it is worth having an emergency plan of additional help which could swing into action during an episode of delirium, if there is no need for hospital treatment. Support and advice are available also from the community dementia team.

If admission to hospital is required, a completed 'This is me' form, downloaded from the Alzheimer's Society website, can be enormously helpful to the staff; it consists of a simple template of facts, likes and dislikes which will help the nurses and may reduce the risk of delirium.

Christian perspectives on dementia

Maintaining our Christian faith in old age and frailty as we cope with the frustration and challenges of disability can be hard, especially if church attendance has become exhausting or impossible. Adding dementia to this can make it even more difficult, where the capacity for concentration and attention is diminished. The church could learn to accommodate, rather than discriminate against, those with failing memory, and many practical materials and publications have been produced to assist church leaders in running church services which are truly accessible to those with mental health issues.

There is a risk of regarding Christian faith solely as an act of the mind – that we come to faith through reason and maintain our faith through studying God's word. Yet Jesus showed us that faith is about a relationship with God. Perhaps we have not taken heed of Jesus saying, "Let the little children come to me, and do not hinder them, for the kingdom of God belongs to such as these. Truly I tell you, anyone who will not receive the kingdom of God like a little child will never enter it."[95] God continues to know us intimately regardless of any mental illness, and the Holy Spirit dwells within us. Relationship with God and with others can continue, even though we may be different. The spirit within can be revealed, as my wife observed in a local nursing home when she saw a hairdresser gently minister to someone who had lost all speech through washing her hair and massaging her head. Peace and tranquillity settled in someone who at other times was quite disturbed. You can explore the theology further on this by reading *Finishing Well*[96] and *Dementia: Pastoral Theology and Pastoral Care*[97].

Prayer and prayer ministry may be valuable, for the person and the carer, depending on the situation, to know God's presence and comfort. I witnessed the wonderful ministry of hospital chaplains and their staff sitting beside someone, reciting with them well-known prayers, and leaving a prayer card or perhaps a holding cross. Music therapy often blends with the person's Christian background, as the music centre of our brain is often spared from dementia. Comfort is found in singing familiar hymns as well as well-known songs, and taking part can improve emotions and unlock memories. The mother of a friend of mine was able to sing Welsh hymns right into her last days despite quite severe dementia. 'Singing for the Brain' groups have grown right across the UK. These are all examples of the Holy Spirit connecting with the soul.

Anxiety

Each morning our frailty team gathers the names of patients with suspected frailty who have been admitted to the hospital because of some emergency the previous evening. Some names will crop up repeatedly – one was Ann. The team would decide who was feeling most full of empathy today to listen to Ann.

Ann was a widow living on her own. She had a kind niece who did her shopping and visited several times a week as Ann had no children of her own. Her usual problem was abdominal pain, which had been investigated on a number of occasions in the past with scans and

---

[95] Luke 18:16-17 (NIV)
[96] Ian Knox (2020); *Finishing Well;* SPCK; chapter 12
[97] James Saunders (2002); *Dementia: Pastoral Theology and Pastoral Care;* Grove Books Limited

endoscopies. Sometimes it was chest pain. Her pain would build up, and in the absence of anyone to talk to at home, she would phone NHS Direct who would arrange for a paramedic to assess her, which would lead to hospital again. Each time that I saw her, the pain had settled after a few hours. She would be anxious about what was causing the problem, and I would go through the story and how all the tests this time were normal, just as on previous occasions. I would explain again that the pain seemed to be due to irritable bowel syndrome and sometimes worsened by constipation. We would discuss the pills that can help the pains – unfortunately, there are few medications which ease anxiety without having significant side-effects. I would chat with her niece over the phone, who would sound apologetic that Ann was at the hospital again. Ann's anxiety was longstanding but had worsened since her husband died two years ago. I would listen to Ann and reassure her, but would be conscious that I had little else to offer.

Anxiety is a common companion to frailty. Ann had some loneliness and depression, but her biggest problem was her anxiety. For many older people, the anxiety can be traced back over a lifetime but then intensifies with the impact of frailty. For others, the onset of dementia can trigger anxiety, especially if there is some insight and frustration into the memory difficulty. It is so sad to see all-consuming anxiety at the end of life, when for many the pressures and stresses of life, such as financial worries or employment, are long in the past. Surely old age is meant for peaceful reflection on a life well lived? Anxiety alongside frailty perhaps has four underlying causes: fear, not coping, change and loss of control. Ann was afraid of a disease that had been missed, was not coping with being alone or the changes since losing her husband and moving home, and now felt out of control of her life as well as her symptoms. Listening, understanding and support are probably the best medicines.

Perhaps the comfort we can give is simply that God is with you through it all: "Do not be discouraged, for the LORD your God will be with you wherever you go,"[98] and, "Don't be afraid, for I am with you."[99] Coping with stress is a skill as well as a personality trait; patterns learnt earlier in life are well established and hard to change. Major life changes all come crashing together in frailty and require acceptance at least of the

---

[98] Joshua 1:9 (NIV)
[99] Isaiah, 41:10 (NLT)

things that cannot be unchanged. I love the old Serenity prayer, also popular outside of Christian circles: "God, grant me the serenity to accept the things I cannot change, courage to change the things I can, and *wisdom to know the difference.*" The notion that we are in control of our life is illusory, but modern life tries to convince us otherwise. So much is available at the touch of the computer screen, and in healthcare we start to believe that it is just a matter of finding out what is wrong and then it can be fixed. Jesus follows up the parable of the rich fool with these words: "Who of you by worrying can add a single hour to his life?"[100] Somehow, we must reach a place of acceptance – that frailty and its associated challenges have become part of the journey of life in the present age. But it is so hard for some.

For you to consider

- How might I help someone with their anxiety or low mood?
- Is my church offering to help, and what might make a difference?
- If I am recognising a memory problem, does it need to be named?
- In supporting someone with dementia, can I create an emergency backup plan for a crisis?

---

[100] Luke 12:25 (NIV)

CHAPTER SEVEN

Will She Be Safe?

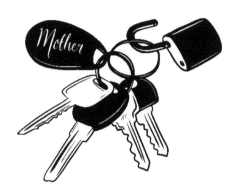

Honour your father and your mother, that your days may be long in the land that the LORD your God is giving you.[101]

ROBERT WAS A MAN OF SEVENTY-NINE YEARS WHOM I remember well as he stayed such a long time on our ward while we discussed his discharge. He had come in with a chest infection which turned out to be pneumonia and took ten days or so to get better. He was old for his years, and rather unkempt. He lived in a council flat in one of the tougher districts of our city, and said he was alone although this turned out not to be entirely true. He was somewhat mal-nourished, but he ate well in hospital and his strength started to return. His skin, hair and nails all benefitted from the loving attention of the nursing staff. After two weeks of treatment, he was well enough to be discharged. However, our social worker then told us that he was an 'adult at risk' and could not be discharged. The police had reported that his house was being used as a drugs den by his son. Robert was evasive about this, saying he was letting his son and other friends use the flat. We also learnt that Robert was giving his pension to his son

---

[101] Exodus 20:12 (ESV)

in exchange for meals and alcohol. There was much discussion as to whether Robert was being abused and if he was happy about all of this. Robert was a little forgetful, but the mental health team and the social worker decided he was capable of making his own decisions. At the end of the day, the police issued a formal warning to the son, and the social worker started once daily care to monitor the situation and left him on the 'adults at risk' register. And Robert went home.

Being discharged from hospital is not usually this complicated, but it is true that for someone living with frailty, there are issues beyond the purely medical ones to be thought through. These can be summarised into two questions:

- Is he safe to be discharged?
- Is she going to manage back at home?

These questions will be as much in the minds of the hospital staff as in the family, the carers, neighbours or anyone else concerned for the welfare of the person. Nine times out of ten, if not ninety-nine times out of a hundred, the person themselves is asking to be allowed home – and if possible, today! Indeed, the motto for our frailty team was "Why not home? Why not today?" to make sure we had a good reason for any other plan. You may think that the hospital just wants to discharge an older person as soon as possible to help cope with the constant pressure of new arrivals each day. While there is undoubtedly some truth in this, there is another side to it: the risks of staying in hospital for someone with frailty are significant (as we have discussed), and hence the desire to discharge is usually in the person's best interests.

Is she going to manage back at home?

Luke the physician is the only Gospel writer who recounts Jesus' beautiful story of the Good Samaritan. What strikes the geriatrician here is not only the Samaritan's compassion and nursing care, but how he then ensures a 'good discharge' through an all-round care package (in the jargon). He arranges transport by putting him on his own animal; he takes him to a place of safety; he hands over his care to the innkeeper; and he provides financial support to ensure that his ongoing care needs are met. The modern equivalents include hospital transport by Red Cross, who will help to settle the person back at home in the absence of family; assessment and management of risks by the ward team; transfer of care to a community provider; and a financial assessment by a social worker.

I realise that health and social care in the UK today will often fall short of this ideal, but investment in community services particularly to cover the crisis episode has increased substantially over the last twenty years. Indeed, the latest NHS long term plan set a target of April 2021 for local services to be able to respond to acute care needs within two hours in a crisis, and forty-eight hours where the need is a little less urgent.[102] But then COVID struck, and the timescales may well have been set back. I can almost see your wry smile – perhaps trying to find good homecare where you live is very difficult? But this is a political and government issue of adequate funding which we all must press for. How many governments have promised to fix proper social care funding for our ageing population?

Managing back at home depends on whether the illness and the admission have affected the person's independence and ability to cope. Deconditioning can occur so quickly, especially with the rather passive existence on a hospital ward. Trying to judge whether someone is back to their usual ability to manage is fraught with difficulty in hospital because nothing is quite the same. Our therapists can make some sort of judgement, but I have often heard the therapist saying they can manage to toilet themselves independently, yet at home in their own bathroom it was going to be far more of a challenge. Or vice versa – they could not really manage in the hospital, but with the familiar arrangement of rails, something to hold onto, and furniture at home, they had their special albeit risky way of doing it. The best way a discharge can be facilitated is by someone from the family or another carer coming into the hospital and discussing with the therapist or discharge coordinator, and helping us understand just how it works, or doesn't work, at home. Get involved as soon as possible; you will be welcomed with open arms. Where there is continuing doubt, a home visit can be requested. And allowance must be made for some improvement once back at home.

Your concern, if you are a carer or family member, may be that she was not managing at home very well before this admission. It is good to describe those concerns to the hospital staff, ideally to whoever is acting

---

[102] NHS Long Term Plan (2018); NHS Long Term Plan » 1. We will boost 'out-of-hospital' care, and finally dissolve the historic divide between primary and community health services

as the discharge coordinator. So often there has been reluctance, or indeed refusal, to admit to the need for help until the present crisis, but now there may be a change of heart and a spot of realism. One common way round this is for the hospital to arrange short term support, which is free and can be a taster as well as a time of assessment. This is called 'reablement'. The absence of cost can help persuade some to accept the offer. If you are sure that continued care after discharge will be needed, and if you believe they would be liable to pay for this, you can go ahead and organise it straight away; I am amazed how many people think they must go through social services, when it may be far quicker to organise yourself at a similar cost and avoid all the waiting.

Is he safe to be discharged?

Sometimes a doctor may paternalistically, or indeed judgementally, pronounce, "Not safe for discharge," or, "He can never be left on his own again," perhaps because they were appalled at how someone had neglected themselves or kept falling at home. Likewise, a junior therapist unfamiliar with the risky lives led by so many older people may pronounce, "Unsafe." Carers and family are quite rightly concerned about the risks of someone living with frailty at home, and the recent crisis has added to those concerns. Perhaps you have been the one saying, "Not safe for discharge," with concerns such as the risk of falling and being stuck on the floor, or the risk of forgetting to take tablets, or not eating and drinking enough? Yet as a Christian you are keen to respect the wishes of an older person to struggle on at home. Can we be justified in imposing our choice?

We must remember that older people living with frailty are used to risk. So, what do we mean by 'not safe'? What is 'safe enough'? The question might be better phrased, "Would she be safer at home?" as hospital living is not very safe either. Nowhere is without risks, but there will be times when moving to live somewhere else is the best and right choice. Being safe enough to go home is always going to be a subjective rather than objective decision and influenced by everyone's acceptance of risk.

If the decision is to go home, then the challenge is to reduce the risks as far as possible through the use of care and home adaptations. Alarm systems have evolved into Telecare – a range of technology solutions and gadgets to assist living, particularly for those with dementia. They include automatic light switches on rising from bed, talking pill dispensers, falls bracelets, smoke detectors, ambient temperature monitors and door alarms triggered on leaving the house at night. The technology probably knows no limits. All devices are monitored through a central control system which can alert family or carers. The Local Authority will have a contract with one company who will assess and give advice. I have seen notable success with door alarms for someone with dementia previously wandering the streets at night, but controlled research trials have not yet shown that assistive technology delays admission to nursing homes.[103] More debatable is the use of cameras to monitor – you might choose to install these, but I would be concerned about whether this is a justifiable intrusion into privacy.

Should I become my parents' carer?

As a hospital doctor, I appreciated when families volunteered to sort out all the care for my patient after discharge. Christians are very conscious of the Fifth Commandment to "honour your father and mother". If we respect their decision to go home, and perhaps without social care, may we feel pressurised to become their carer? Or do we feel guilty in refusing?

Ann Benton in her utterly practical book *If It's Not Too Much Trouble*[104] describes a methodical approach to assessing whether and how you should become more involved. She advises first to assess the need – is it emotional, practical or physical? – and then figure out what you can offer. My wife's mother lived more than two hours away, and my wife would visit every month as her mother became more disabled and began to fall. She needed some hands-on care, but also a huge amount of reassurance as she became increasingly anxious. My wife is an only child, so this increased the pressure to become the carer, but their relationship worked best at an emotional and physical distance. The need was for someone to be present every day, and my wife recognised that this would put too much strain on their relationship, and hands-on care would be challenging. Thinking this through helped to reduce a sense of guilt.

---

[103] Howard R *et al* (2021); 'The effectiveness and cost-effectiveness of assistive technology and telecare for independent living in dementia: A randomised controlled trial'; Age Ageing 50, Issue 3, May 2021; pp.882-890

[104] Benton Ann (2007); *If It's Not Too Much Trouble;* Christian Focus

Matthew Henry's commentary on the Fifth Commandment includes "endeavouring in everything to be the comfort of their old age and to make their old age easy for them"[105]. Paul wrote to the young Timothy advising him how to ensure that the local church was providing for their widows correctly: "But if she has children or grandchildren, these should learn first of all to put their religion into practice by caring for their own family."[106] This seems like a clear instruction – but the Greek word can be translated 'provide' and has the sense of 'plan before'. There is the sense of taking responsibility and planning here, ensuring that good care is provided, and in that way not leaving it to the church to provide.

Jesus gives the ultimate example of taking responsibility for planning good care for his mother. As He hangs on the cross, He commissions the disciple John to take care of her. Another illustration is when Jesus sees the funeral cortege for an only son of a widow – "His heart overflowed with compassion."[107] And with the authority Jesus has over death, He commands the man back to life. I believe we have the instructions here to honour our parents by planning and ensuring they are well provided for, but this may not be the same as becoming their carer. As a health professional, I would never seek to influence these difficult family decisions, nor make any judgements.

It can be a beautiful thing where family are indeed able to provide care, and relationships are strengthened rather than stretched to the limit. Living with frailty can be hard, and caring for those who are living with frailty can equally be demanding. But there can be mutual fulfilment in the work of caring for each other. In God's world, growth often occurs through a time of adversity, and God can be particularly close during those times in our life, even if it does not feel like that. This was expressed by Jesus in the beatitudes:

> *Blessed are the poor in spirit, for theirs is the kingdom of heaven.*
> *Blessed are those who mourn, for they will be comforted.*
> *Blessed are the meek, for they will inherit the earth.*[108]

---

[105] *Matthew Henry Bible Commentary* (complete); Exodus 20; christianity.com
[106] 1 Timothy 5:4 (NIV)
[107] Luke 7:13 (NLT)
[108] Matthew 5:3-5 (NIV)

If you are the partner of the person needing support, hopefully you will accept outside help as well. I often met partners who had become dissatisfied by the standard of care being provided by external carers – perhaps arriving unreliably or being a little brusque – and had then cancelled the care completely. This can easily precipitate exhaustion. Over the years I met hundreds of carers who had been stretched to the limit and would blame other members of the family for not playing their part, or social services for not responding when asked. And such stress brings dangers. Ann Benton describes when goodwill, peace of mind and joy in serving are lost, with the consequences of a bad temper, bitterness, walking out, blaming and even violence.[109]

Most elder abuse is perpetrated by those intimately involved in the care of the older person – abuse such as verbal abuse, neglect, financial abuse or even physical abuse. Most of the abuse I met as a consultant arose within the context of love mixed with duty. Recognising when you as a carer are near breaking point, or perhaps past breaking point, is important. It is best to have some regular help to share the load and give yourself time off. There is the danger that guilt might drive you to go beyond what you can reasonably manage, and this can trigger unintended abuse. The apostle Paul wrote, "No testing has overtaken you that is not common to everyone. God is faithful, and he will not let you be tested beyond your strength, but with the testing he will also provide the way out so that you may be able to endure it."[110] But it may not seem like this. The truth is that there are always places to turn to, as you look for the "way out" God has provided. Unfortunately, on many occasions I encountered someone brought to the hospital ED ostensibly because of a medical symptom, and then the family would tell me they refused to have them back home as they could not cope any longer. The hospital should not be used in this way, but it can be the place of last resort. Sometimes, after a few days of a break in caring, and when symptoms or behaviour have settled somewhat, the partner or family would feel they could manage again, perhaps with increased care support. Social services run an 'Adults At Risk' helpline which provides urgent help and advice for these situations.

---

[109] Benton Ann (2007); *If It's Not Too Much Trouble;* Christian Focus
[110] 1 Corinthians 10:13 (NRSV)

Whom to believe?

Our elderly assessment team met Judith, who came into hospital following a fall at home. She was eighty-five and lived alone, fiercely independent but having some support from her daughter. A GP summary on the IT system detailed her diagnoses of dementia and previous breast cancer. She had extensive body scans because of bruising and the fall, and this revealed that Judith now had widespread secondary cancer.

We discussed the findings with Judith as we considered that she could understand the results in spite of her dementia – she was very convincing. She wanted to go home and felt she was currently managing well, saying she had just tripped over her dog.

We were about to discharge her but talked this over with her daughter. She told us about Judith's symptoms of pain and breathlessness (not divulged by Judith) and frequent panic phone calls yet refusing any outside help. Her daughter wanted to arrange some respite care for Judith to be looked after, to see how things went. A lasting power of attorney was in process but not yet activated. We relayed this to Judith later in the day, who was very cross with her daughter but also more confused, not recalling our conversations of the morning. It became clear that she lacked insight into her present and future situation regarding both her disease and managing at home. We therefore agreed with the daughter's plan for respite care and assisted her daughter in making the arrangements for the following day. We contacted the nursing home to hand over her care.

Judith illustrated the benefits of specialist assessment soon after admission, and involvement of the family. Our team initially thought we should facilitate Judith's wishes for discharge back home, given that she had a limited outlook of weeks, or at best months, left to live. The whole situation was far from ideal, and the desire to avoid a protracted admission to hospital led to a hurried move into respite care. But Judith's dementia, along with her reluctance to admit to the true implications of her diagnosis, nearly led us to create further problems through an unwise discharge home.

"I always promised Mum she would never go to a nursing home." This may have been a kind but reckless promise years ago, but hard to forget. The Bible has some interesting instructions about vows. Jesus had an argument with some Pharisees which started as a dispute about his disciples not following their traditions. But Jesus then countered that they had used the vow of Corban to avoid their duty to provide for their parents.[111] The vow of Corban was a trick used by some Pharisees – they would allocate some of their resources to the temple, meaning that 'Corban' money was not available to fund their parents' care. And apparently, they would still have access to that 'restricted fund' anyway. So, the vow of Corban was a ruse, stopping them doing the right thing. Perhaps similarly, we should be aware of being held by past vows. Jesus said, "Again, you have heard that it was said to the people long ago, 'Do not break your oath, but fulfil to the Lord the vows you have made.' But I tell you, do not make any vows! ... All you need to say is simply 'Yes' or 'No'; anything beyond this comes from the evil one."[112] God's love for us is not dependent on whether we have kept promises made in the past – thankfully, there is forgiveness by the grace of God. We need to be honest to ourselves and others about what we can do or commit to.

There is a danger of taking advantage of a person's vulnerability while in hospital and imposing a degree of control over them which might have been impossible at home. This arguably happened for Judith. Yet for some this may also be the moment when realism has struck home, and an acceptance of the need for help follows. A balance between respecting autonomy and a paternalistic behaviour (or is this reverse paternalism, as we make decisions for our parents, rather than they for us?) is needed. Honouring our parents may justify paternalism on occasion. But it is good to remember that taking risk is vital to the human spirit. So hopefully, a joint person-centred discussion can take place to reach an agreed way forward. Where there is a degree of dementia or other mental health disorder, a lasting power of attorney for health and welfare is intended to enable the attorney to act on the person's behalf in these decisions, and this should reduce any feelings of guilt. However, this only authorises the attorney to communicate and respect the decision the person would have made for themselves if they were back in their own usual sound mind. This can be difficult and sometimes pragmatism must prevail, as illustrated here with Judith.

For my wife's mother, her care needs increased, and a series of live-in carers proved unsettling and unsatisfactory. This, combined with frequent falling, led to a decision to move her into a care home close to

---

[111] Mark 7:11 (NIV)
[112] Matthew 5:33-37 (NIV)

where we lived. This seemed an ideal situation – her daily physical and reassurance needs were met, there was always someone around to help her at the care home, and my wife was able to visit regularly.

Finding the right care home

I think you will know when you visit a care home if it feels like a place in which your relative could feel at home. You will be looking to find kindness and love in the staff you meet, and homeliness and personal effects in residents' rooms. It is probably rather less about efficiency and procedures, although it is important that these things are running properly in the background. The Care Quality Commission ratings for every registered home are available on the internet and are worth looking at but do tend to emphasise adherence to those procedures as well as staff training rather than the 'feel' of the place. Do you see happy faces as you look around? If possible, talk to someone who has had a relative in that care home. You may be interested to explore The Pilgrim Friends Society which currently run eleven dementia care homes with a Christian ethos, and many care homes have a church or Christian foundation under-pinning them.

My medical advice is to ensure the home has a regular GP visit, ideally every week. It makes a great difference to the staff to have reliable support, and this will reduce the need for future hospital visits.

When falling begins

Decisions about risks at home, or moving into care, are often influenced by the risk of further falls and what might happen. Falling becomes commonplace as we age because our balance and strength deteriorate. Try standing on one leg with your eyes closed for twenty seconds! Around a third to a half of those living with moderate frailty will have multiple falls every year. Here is a checklist we can work through; these can reduce the frequency of falls, but probably not stop them altogether:

- If a walking aid inside the house is needed to maintain balance, make sure it is used every time. I must have seen hundreds of patients in the emergency department who had just forgotten to use their aid that day. A therapy review confirmed that they were safe if using the aid. But this is a greater problem for those with memory impairment.

- If living alone, rent a falls alarm system – available from the local council but usually needs a telephone line. They only work if worn at all times – again, how many times have I been told, "Oh, I always take it off at night," when they had fallen going to the toilet at night and spent the rest of the night on the floor.
- Arrange a medication review, as discussed before.
- Arrange an optician appointment to review sight and glasses.
- Look out for trip hazards around the house.
- Arrange a chiropody appointment, and wear comfortable shoes, not those poor-fitting slippers.
- Ask the GP about a referral to a falls clinic for a review of possible causes for the falling. Amongst other things, they will want to check blood pressure when lying and standing – a drop on standing is a common cause for losing balance.
- Keep active and participate in exercise classes if possible.

After taking these steps, it is important to recognise that falls cannot be stopped altogether. Those living with frailty live with that risk. To use St Paul's words rather out of context, "...and after you have done everything, to stand. Stand firm then..."[113] In other words, accept that some falls will still happen – and taking to bed is not the answer either. It can be harder for the family to live with the knowledge that falls may happen when no-one is around than it is for the person themselves. Falls will continue in a care home but at least someone to help will be close at hand when the fall does happen.

Going back to hospital again

Sometimes being back home just does not work out. The planned support was not enough, the falls kept happening, the symptoms returned or the confusion worsened. Reflecting on this, the support can be adjusted, the home made a little safer and the medication adjusted again. This is a familiar cycle for those living with frailty. But the crises keep coming. It is very tempting to think that the hospital just did not get to the bottom of it all – surely, there must be a reason for this pain or

---

[113] Ephesians 6:13-14 (NIV)

weakness or dizziness? This is quite unlike any sort of malingering or hypochondriasis. But fixing one or two parts is just not enough to restore health. Indeed, very quickly a cycle is begun of diminishing returns. Longer or recurrent spells in hospital take their toll, with all the adverse events associated with a hospital stay we discussed in chapter five. Even if a second or third admission does identify a hidden diagnosis which might be the answer, it is very hard to translate this into successful treatment and rehabilitation for those with marked frailty – it is a high mountain to climb – although it happens for some. There comes a time when it is better to be pragmatic and focus on managing the symptoms. This equates to acceptance. This may sound rather negative – but the time for acceptance will be different for everyone, and you will probably know in your heart when further hospitalisation is not the answer. It is a step on the road to letting go. It may even be putting your trust in God rather than in healthcare.

For you to consider

- Make sure you get involved in discharge planning early on.
- If you are a carer, do you need to ask for more help? How could you give yourself a break?
- Decision-making for those with dementia is more complex, to strike the right balance between respecting individual choice and ensuring good care, and feelings of guilt are common. Why not talk this through with your church leader?
- If falls are happening, have you worked through a checklist like this?

CHAPTER EIGHT

Planning Ahead

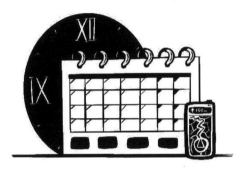

Teach us to realise the brevity of life, so that we may grow in wisdom.[114]

CHARLIE WAS AN EIGHTY-NINE-YEAR-OLD GENTLEMAN who was referred to the community matron by the practice nurse because she felt "this normally dapper chap was looking a bit dowdy" and she wondered if he and his wife were not coping. He had a complex medical history, with heart failure and chronic lung disease, and was entirely reliant upon continuous oxygen therapy. His life was very limited by shortness of breath and fatigue.

A home assessment was carried out and it was obvious that control was paramount to Charlie; after all, he had run some of the biggest companies in the world and he described himself as the "ultimate wheeler dealer". Initially he was rather cagey, preferring to say that they were managing well. However, his wife of sixty years set the record straight, highlighting his extreme shortness of breath, and exhaustion. As she described it, their once vibrant international lifestyle was limited to "life at the end of the tube". She also confided

---

[114] Psalm 90:12 (NLT)

that they were both getting on each other's nerves – something they were sad about as they remained very much in love.

Over a couple of visits, a self-management supportive plan was jointly devised. This included a home oxygen review, help from physiotherapy, occupational therapy and a visit from me for medication review. All this allowed Charlie to manage his breathlessness better and he was able to get into his garden to feel "the sunshine on his face" which was very important both to him and his wife.

After three good months, he called urgently for help. A home visit revealed he was ill and possibly nearing death. An advance care plan had already been completed but Charlie wanted to add "NO HOSPITAL, NO EXCEPTIONS". He was terrified about being a burden to his wife and family whilst acknowledging that he was "knackered, clapped out and past his sell-by date". He confided he hated being out of control and reliant upon his wife and family. A family discussion took place, and it was clear that Charlie would be cared for at home by his family with the support of the community matron and district nursing team. End of life drugs were prescribed, along with glasses of French wine and other favoured 'tipples'! Two days later Charlie died at home, surrounded by his family.

Are you good at decisions or do you put things off? We are all made differently, and some of those personality traits can be revealed by profiles such as the Myers Briggs Personality Test.[115] The fourth dimension of the Myers Briggs is labelled 'perceiving or judging'. 'Perceiving' types go with the flow and enjoy flexibility and spontaneity when it comes to agendas or decisions. 'Judging' types take an organised approach to life, and prefer that future events be planned out or scheduled to go as smoothly as possible. Thankfully, my wife and I are both of the 'judging' type which means we like planning ahead. In the UK, a recent survey found that sixty percent of adults had not made a will, and this figure was increasing rather than decreasing.[116] If you are more the 'perceiving' type, you may put off making decisions such as writing a will and feel you can do it another day – after all, you are perfectly well at the moment. No-one likes talking about death, and especially their own.

---

[115] Myers Briggs personality assessment instrument; The Myers & Briggs Foundation – Take the MBTI® Instrument; accessed 27.12.2020

[116] 'Over half (60%) of UK adults don't have a will'; yourmoney.com

Much of this book has been about patient-centred care, and how to enable us to be fully involved in decisions about our own health or the healthcare of family members or a close friend. Unfortunately, when big decisions are required, that moment is frequently when we, or our nearest and dearest, are most distressed and least able to be actively involved in any decision. We may just be too ill. Imagine Charlie's situation with no advance care plan. He might have struggled to the toilet in the night in those last weeks and collapsed out of breath. A phone call for emergency help brought the paramedics, who, in their proficient and professional manner, took over with reassuring confidence. In the absence of any clear advance care plan, the paramedics would be duty-bound to resuscitate him and race him off to hospital. He would never make it back home. Many people think like Charlie, wanting to remain in control and embarrassed at the thought of being out of control.

Two of the barriers to completing a living will, known in the UK as an advance care plan, are inertia and ignorance of how to do it. Another barrier can come from the family not listening – Kathryn Mannix explains:

> *This conspiracy of silence is so common, and so heartbreaking. The elderly expect death, and many try to talk to others about their hopes and wishes. But often they are rebuffed by the young, who cannot bear, or even contemplate, those thoughts that are the constant companions of the aged or the sick.*[117]

Baroness Neuberger, in her book *Not Dead Yet*[118], reflected on the interviews she had carried out before writing her book:

> *Most of the older people I know seem remarkably unscared of dying. ... There is no doubt that older people know death is coming, and their fear is very often not so much of death itself, but of being warehoused in a hospital that can do little for them, or a nursing home where they will be expected to sit still and wait.*

[117] Kathryn Mannix (2017); *With the End in Mind: Dying, Death and Wisdom in an Age of Denial;* p.127; HarperCollins
[118] Julia Neuberger (2008); *Not Dead Yet;* p.281; Harper Collins

How much truer has this been during the year of COVID, with enforced restrictions on family support in hospital or care homes. Choices between what we valued most were taken out of our hands to protect the lives of the most vulnerable – autonomy was lost.

Seeing it coming

None of us can know how long we have to live, and this is certainly true for those living with frailty, where changes in health can be very gradual. We don't like being honest about the seriousness of our health problems. As a consultant for older people, I witnessed the whole spectrum of insight when I was explaining someone's health outlook to them. Some would appreciate their situation, and my conversation with them would simply be confirming their own thoughts and suspicions. At the other end of the spectrum, there would be complete denial of any problems, perhaps because they had lived with these problems for so long, and this would make it much harder for me to be frank, and risked appearing uncaring. My own natural style was to be honest and straight-talking, and I found that this was appreciated by many older people who had lived with frailty and the prospect of the end of their life for some years. Charlie was initially reluctant to face up to the reality of his situation, but when a good relationship had been formed with the community matron over a few weeks, this allowed patient-centred care and a care plan which satisfied Charlie and his wife. Coming to terms with all of this creates a window of opportunity to establish our wishes for future medical treatment, given the distinct possibility that when the time comes, we may lack the mental capacity to explain our wishes ourselves.

Who is in control?

Medical treatment must be given with the consent of the patient, and that consent is legally defined – we must be able to understand what is being proposed, understand the risks and be able to communicate our understanding and agreement to proceed. If we can do all that, we are judged to have 'mental capacity' for the decision in hand. Someone who has mental capacity can legally refuse to have any more treatment, even if this means their life will end as a result. This principle becomes more opaque in dealing with emergencies, where there is presumed consent even if the person at that moment has lost mental capacity because, for example, an ambulance was called to help.

As a Christian, refusing a treatment which could save our life may pose a problem, feeling that life is God-given and that we should not make any 'life and death' decision for ourselves. We do not need to 'allow things to take their course' when medicine can be lifesaving. We trust that ultimately God is in control, but equally we may feel uneasy at our doctors 'playing God' by giving treatments which may be postponing a natural death. Living gracefully with frailty may involve letting go of control to those who care for us – this was beautifully described by Wanda Nash in her book *Come Let Us Age!*[119]:

> *Whether we are ever 'in control' is a debatable matter, but certainly the feeling of losing control is extremely debilitating and can feel humiliating. So, let's give control away, rather than fretting that it is being snatched from us.*

In one sense, none of us are in control – we can only make decisions. Doctors know only too well that events take their own course, and there are constant surprises. In addition, Christians may not want to overemphasise autonomy in the modern sense of being 'all about me', but rather to be aware that any decision they make impacts on others. Reflecting on the humility of Christ, the apostle Paul said, "Each of you should look not only to your own interests, but also to the interests of others."[120] I have met many long-suffering patients who have said to me, "But I must keep going for my husband's sake," conscious of the grief their own death would cause to the ones they love.

For those living with frailty or dementia, a severe illness which takes them to hospital will commonly cause a delirium, robbing them of mental capacity and reducing their chance of being able to refuse a treatment. If we are unable to consent, then the doctor will act in what they believe to be in our best interests and give any treatment which has a reasonable chance of being 'successful'. Unfortunately, this creates a significant grey area where treatments are being given which may well succeed in prolonging life a little longer, but where there is little chance of real recovery.

---

[119] Nash, Wanda (2017); *Come, Let Us Age!;* Bible Reading Fellowship; p.32
[120] Philemon 2:4 (NIV)

Recording our wishes and preferences in advance

If in Wanda Nash's words, we wish to "give control away", there are two legal mechanisms for recording our future wishes regarding our medical treatment. One is by appointing an Attorney for Health and Welfare; the other is by drawing up an advance care plan or 'living will'. A survey of British attitudes in 2013 revealed the status of living wills.[121] Although seventy percent claimed to be comfortable talking about death, and two-thirds had experienced bereavement in the previous five years, "Only 5% had made an advance care plan setting out how they would want to be cared for if they couldn't make decisions themselves. Although the latest NHS figures show that more than half of people currently die in hospital, only 7% of respondents to the survey said they would prefer to die in hospital, with more than two thirds (sixty-seven percent) saying that they would prefer to die at home."

A lasting power of attorney (LPA) for health and welfare is a similar document to a lasting power of attorney for financial affairs, and often a solicitor will suggest we complete both at the same time. The LPA must be registered by the solicitor with the Court of Protection, and a cost is involved. Essentially, we are asking a close relative or friend in whom we trust to make decisions on our behalf if we are unable to do so. This should mean ideally that we have been prepared to discuss with them how we feel about having certain treatments towards the end of life, so their decisions do indeed reflect our own opinions. We may wish to refuse certain treatments even if this means our life will end. Arguably the greatest benefit from these documents is those conversations. This will be tough and stressful, trying to imagine possible future scenarios. There are probably all sorts of scenarios we would never think of, so including our GP in the discussion will be very helpful. Hopefully, the fear for the future may be softened a little by our trust in our relative to make wise decisions on our behalf. The attorney may still have agonisingly difficult decisions to face in the future, mixed with guilt, but remembering those conversations will provide reassurance that they are doing the right thing.

The alternative is to complete an advance decision to refuse treatment (ADRT), which is defined in law by the Mental Capacity Act

---

[121] British Social Attitudes survey 30 (2013); 'Dying';
https://www.bsa.natcen.ac.uk/media/38850/bsa_30_dying.pdf

enacted in 2005. If we want our views to be legally binding, then we must have followed the exact procedure detailed in the Act:

- We are aged eighteen or over and have the capacity to make, understand and communicate our decision.
- We clearly specify which treatments we wish to refuse, even if this could lead to our death.
- We explain the circumstances in which we wish to refuse them.
- It is signed and witnessed.
- We have made the decision of our own accord.
- We have not said anything since making the advance decision to indicate we have changed our mind.

There are several ADRT forms which can be downloaded from the internet, for example from Compassion in Dying[122] and Macmillan Cancer Support[123]. They are best completed again during a conversation with our own doctor, with a family member present to act as our witness. Copies of the completed ADRT will be kept by us and our doctor. It can of course be reviewed at any time and updated as we wish, keeping our GP informed. One difficulty with an ADRT is trying to anticipate the precise situation we might be in during a crisis; the attending doctor in the crisis may feel we had not foreseen the situation and feel obliged to give life-saving treatment, even if this might not have been our wish. It is important to understand that an advance care plan cannot insist on being given any specific treatment. Doctors cannot be forced to give a treatment which they feel has no chance of being of benefit to the person. Likewise, an advance care plan cannot instruct a doctor to end our life – it does not permit physician-assisted suicide, the active provision of a medicine given with the intention that the patient will use it to end their life.

Another approach has been the introduction of the RESPECT form by the Resuscitation Council in the UK in 2016.[124] Its increasingly widespread (but not yet universal) use across the UK is improving familiarity for health professionals. This form records our wishes for future treatment without being legally enforceable. It stands for Recommended Summary Plan for Emergency Care and Treatment. A

---

[122] https://compassionindying.org.uk/library/advance-decision-pack
[123] https://www.macmillan.org.uk/_images/ADRTDocument_20170505_JS_tcm9-311758.pdf
[124] www.resus.org.uk/respect

clearly completed RESPECT form, combined perhaps with our relative confirming what we have expressed in previous conversations, should enable our wishes to be respected. It does help if the statements are precise, and hence the importance of completing this form with our GP. Vague statements like "To be treated at home if possible" are unlikely to alter the decisions made by paramedic staff when attending in an emergency, who never transfer patients to hospital unless necessary. Mildred's RESPECT form (chapter four) was rather vague and permitted the paramedics to refer her to the hospital to be treated. Charlie's RESPECT form was very direct: "NO HOSPITAL, NO EXCEPTIONS". Here are some other precise examples:

- Home/community is preferred location for care, with admission to hospital only to be considered if symptoms are unmanageable in the community.
- Hospital admission is to be avoided at all costs; patient very clear they do not wish to be admitted, even if this will result in death.
- Hospital admission only for probable fracture but consider period of observation and GP review prior to transfer to hospital. Not for hospital otherwise, even if this will result in death.

The RESPECT form has a section to indicate our preferences on what we feel will matter most to us towards the end of life. This is sometimes called an advance statement. We might include:

- foods we do and don't like;
- what kind of clothes we prefer to wear;
- the type of music we like and what we like to watch on TV;
- whether we like to sleep with a light on;
- our religious or other beliefs and values;
- who we would like to visit us.

For a thorough introduction to the practicalities of making a living will, you can read *Time To Live* by Ann Clifford[125] which gives much more detail on many aspects of facing our mortality and planning ahead. You can also look at the Age UK website.[126]

---

[125] Clifford, Ann (2017); *Time To Live;* Instant Apostle
[126] Age UK (April 2020); 'Factsheet 72 Advance decisions, advance statements and living wills'; ageuk.org.uk

A Christian viewpoint

There are mixed views amongst Christians regarding making decisions to refuse treatments ahead of time. For some it seems too close to euthanasia – making a personal choice about when life has nothing more to offer. Surely God continues to see us as valuable and pours His love on us, regardless of our degree of dependency? Can we say when life no longer has meaning? Also, it is impossible to know how we will feel when experiencing illness or disability; the healthy do not choose in the same way as the sick. Life will seem more precious when we have less of it. My wife and I knew an older lady, already somewhat frail and disabled, who became quadriplegic after a car accident. When we visited her some weeks after the accident, she said she no longer wished to live with such severe disability. She put it like this: "I think it's time I made my exit." However, she came to terms with the situation and found some meaning for life. She did not face any life-threatening illness and lived some years in a care home with amazing fortitude and a strong Christian faith.

In dementia such as Alzheimer's disease, there will be come a time when mental capacity is lost, when it would be too late to instruct an LPA. This needs to be drawn up possibly years, or at least months, before it is needed. It is even more difficult to imagine how we would feel about our quality of life and our wishes for life-saving treatments when in advanced dementia. We can choose to whom we hand over control, and I believe that many of us will derive more comfort from handing control to one we love and trust through an LPA, rather than leaving this to a doctor. It will still be very hard for our attorney to know when the time has come to refuse any life-saving treatment on our behalf, partly because the changes may be so gradual.

In some ways, the introduction and legalisation of advance care plans shows the public's mistrust of doctors to act always in the patient's best interests, and the medical profession's tendency to fight to prolong life regardless of the consequences. This is the fear of being kept alive on a machine. In practice this is less of an issue in caring for those with severe frailty because intensive life support is less likely to be offered by the doctors and is more likely to be futile in terms of successfully restoring life. Nevertheless, it remains a fear for many.

The Christian Medical Fellowship has had ambivalence regarding advance care plans, and has previously expressed what they feel is a better way:[127]

> *But there comes a time in the life of every patient when these options are closed, and treatment would be worse than useless. When that stage is reached, the easing of death should be seen as a positive achievement. Futile treatment and the prolongation of dying should be viewed as a serious failure of care. If therapy is withheld as being inappropriate, such action must not be condemned as 'playing God'. The withholding of treatment is no more 'playing God' than is the institution of treatment. Neither action ensures the outcome. The consultant has the responsibility of discussing the matter fully with the caring team and explaining the reasoning behind any decision not to treat or resuscitate.*

My own view is that advance care plans and RESPECT have a valuable place to play in the healthcare of those living with frailty and nearing the end of life, alongside a trusting relationship with our local healthcare team. Fear of the dying process, rather than fear of death, is natural for all of us, no matter how strong our belief in the journey after death. For some, this fear can be reduced by trusting someone else to act on our behalf. I have witnessed too many times that a person was unable to die at home in comfort and at peace, with their family around them as they had wished, because in the moment of an emergency with urgent medical need, that medical need was met by coming into hospital. The symptoms could usually be managed at home, assisted by the GP, the community nursing service, and supported as needed by the Macmillan service and specialist palliative care staff. Where this has been discussed and agreed before, there is a better chance of this happening.

Cardiac resuscitation

One element in these conversations will be wishes regarding resuscitation. When talking to patients or their family, I would usually raise the question as to whether this has ever been discussed. The reply some of the time would be along the lines, "Oh, yes, she has said she

---

[127] Short, D (1993); Euthanasia Booklet *Should Doctors Support the Living Will?;* Christian Medical Fellowship; chapter 4

doesn't want any resuscitation," although most times this would not have been written down anywhere, or on a signed document, so carried no legal weight.

Let's briefly think through the practicalities of resuscitation. The full title, at least in this context, is cardiopulmonary resuscitation (CPR), and it is usually discussed in the context of a sudden catastrophic illness in the heart or lungs. And of course, a heart attack is by far the most common cause. Most people will have seen a cardiac arrest on the TV, either a real-life arrest or in a TV soap. Successful resuscitation in real life is less common than on the TV; a survey of American TV soaps found sixty cases of attempted CPR, with success in three quarters.[128] In the UK there are around one hundred thousand heart attacks a year coming to hospital, and around thirty thousand cardiac arrests outside of hospital. The chance of surviving outside of hospital is about one in ten.[129] If the cardiac arrest occurs in hospital there is a slightly better chance of surviving, mainly because of the immediate availability of resuscitation. However, the survival chances for people over the aged of eighty are about half of this, and then even lower if the person has other illnesses as well.[130] If the person has any cancer or chronic lung disease or kidney failure, for example, this worsens the chance of survival. Where there is moderate or advanced frailty, the chance of survival falls to two percent or less.[131]

In a cardiac arrest, the heart has stopped beating effectively. After initial chest compressions, an electric shock to the chest must be given to restart the heart. If this is successful, the person will require intensive support over the next few days. If breathing has also stopped, then they may well require to be ventilated for a few days in an intensive care unit. The whole process is traumatic and sometimes rather gruesome. It is not a dignified departure for those who do not survive. For all these reasons, doctors will encourage someone living with frailty to accept the idea of

---

[128] Diem S, Lantos J, Tulsky J (1996); 'Cardiopulmonary Resuscitation on Television'; NEJM 334:1578-82

[129] Resuscitation Council (2013); 'Consensus Paper on Out-of-Hospital Cardiac Arrest in England'; OHCA_consensus_paper.pdf (resus.org.uk)

[130] Mike S van Gijn et al (2014); 'The chance of survival and the functional outcome after in-hospital cardiopulmonary resuscitation in older people: a systematic review'; Age and Ageing 43.456-463

[131] Ibitoye S et al (2020); 'Frailty status predicts futility of cardiopulmonary resuscitation in older adults'; Age Ageing 50 (1) 147-152

not attempting CPR. In my experience, the majority of older people believe this themselves, almost intuitively, without necessarily knowing the statistics. They are comfortable with the notion that if their heart stops, then their time has come. Indeed, this is partly why the abbreviation to summarise this advanced decision is shifting from DNACPR – 'do not attempt cardiopulmonary resuscitation' – to AND – 'allow natural death'.

Views in the Jewish community

But not everyone has the same viewpoint. I remember treating a Jewish patient who was severely ill from heart failure. His family observed Halacha, traditional Jewish law, which governs every aspect of Jewish life and ethics. Halacha deems that life is of infinite value, and therefore the imperative to preserve life supersedes every other consideration.[132] In my opinion, attempted CPR was certain to fail in his case, and would probably add to the distress at the end of his life, which I anticipated was only a few days away at best. The large team needed for CPR must surround the patient and ask the family to move outside of the room while they give some quite aggressive treatments. So, the family are separated just as life is slipping away. This family was insistent that resuscitation should be attempted. Only a few days later our resuscitation team indeed had to try CPR when his heart stopped – and the family were grateful for all we had done including our attempts to resuscitate. Jewish law has now suggested a distinction should be drawn between ordinary medical treatment (for example, fluids, antibiotics, surgery) and extraordinary treatment (which would include CPR and ventilators), and Jews are permitted to refuse CPR.

Some Christians may also feel that a 'do not resuscitate' order is morally wrong, disrespecting the sanctity of life, as God has ordained when life ends: "...all the days ordained for me were written in your book before one of them came to be,"[133] and, "Since their days are determined, and the number of their months is known to you, and you have appointed the bounds that they cannot pass."[134] In the context of advanced frailty,

---

[132] Rabbi Schostak (1994); 'Jewish ethical guidelines for resuscitation and artificial nutrition and hydration of the dying elderly'; Journal of Medical Ethics 20: 93-100

[133] Psalm 139:16 (NIV)

[134] Job 14:5 (NRSV)

it may be easier to argue that delivering CPR is an attempt to interfere with the natural end of life when the heart has finally stopped beating and God is calling us home.

A movement called 'death cafés' helps people to talk about death and mull over thoughts and preferences over a comforting drink and piece of cake! If you have never thought about all this before, or talked about it with others or your family, it is much harder when confronted by the conversation with a doctor. Why not join a death café in your area? It is amazing how once this conversation has started and the taboo broken, people soon seem to know instinctively what matters most to them.

Can I trust that my wishes will be followed?

Perhaps the greatest benefit of planning ahead and discussing these issues with our family is to bring our hopes and fears into the open. Then when a crisis occurs – as with Charlie – everyone is prepared as well as they can be and our wishes can be respected. However, there can be no guarantee those wishes will be followed: our power of attorney may not be around or available that day; our RESPECT form or advance care plan may not be handed to the doctor or paramedic attending us; or the precise situation might not quite fit with any of the scenarios described in our plans. Indeed, as we would expect, paramedics have clear procedures in relation to life-threatening illness, acute chest pain or suspected stroke which dictate that they 'blue light' transport someone to the hospital immediately, and it may take some cool confidence to dissuade them. In hospital the LPA may only be identified the day after admission, when some emergency treatment has already been given. At that point there can be a full discussion with the attorney about the way ahead if we remain very ill. If the RESPECT form is well-written, it will provide a clear guide to the doctors of our overall wishes for healthcare and will give doctors permission to refrain from any further intrusive treatment.

Our emergency services quite naturally have a default setting to rush in and try to save lives whatever the cost. But there is a strengthening voice asking that our system learns a different response, respecting those who no longer wish their life to be saved in an emergency. The growing familiarity of living wills, RESPECT forms and lasting power of attorney is helping that voice to be heard. The emergency call for help needs to be answered just as urgently but with a light touch – with kindness and medicines to ensure comfort where needed. This is probably better recognised in those dying from cancer, but we need the same understanding of dying with frailty. Perhaps then we will more often witness the dignity of dying at home – as for Charlie.

For you to consider

- Do you feel you should write an advance care plan or complete a RESPECT form? Ask your GP about this.
- Have you appointed a lasting power of attorney for health and welfare?
- Do they need updating?
- If you really want your preferred wishes to be followed, you need to pay attention to detail on the forms.
- You need to make sure the forms are accessible in an emergency, or that the nursing home keep them in a safe place.

CHAPTER NINE

Letting Go

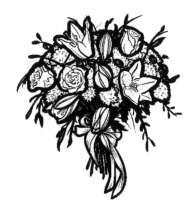

"Sovereign Lord, now let your servant die in peace, as you have promised. I have seen your salvation, which you have prepared for all people."[135]

LETTING GO IS A DRAWN-OUT AFFAIR FOR MOST PEOPLE LIVing with frailty, and many of my patients had already travelled down that road quite a long way by the time we met. It might have begun with letting go of their family home of fifty years, to move nearer a member of their family or perhaps into a retirement flat. It might have involved saying goodbye to treasured possessions and familiar furniture. It might have included letting go of responsibilities at church or volunteering, or perhaps giving up membership of a sports club. And later it might have included asking someone in the family to manage their financial affairs. Others might have refused to let go of anything, and now, after a major stroke or broken hip, had to face the shock of letting go of almost everything all at once. Letting go gracefully can be a release from things we do not need to worry about any longer. This last chapter considers

---

[135] Luke 2:29-31 (NLT)

the final release from a life lived with frailty and considers some of the difficult decisions to be made. Sometimes 'letting go' can only happen when peace takes the place of pain, as shown by Doreen.

Doreen was an eighty-four-year-old widow who was transferred from a nearby community hospital to our hospital to have her leg ulcer assessed. This had been worsening for two months and was giving her intolerable pain. The referring local GP was asking us if we could arrange a surgical opinion. We heard how she had been managing quite well living on her own until six months ago, but her diabetes had worsened, and she fell and injured her leg. The gangrenous ulcer on her shin had not responded to the district nurse's treatments. We were shocked when we met Doreen that afternoon. She looked dreadful and emaciated. As soon as we tried to touch the leg to remove the dressing and examine her, she was shouting out in pain. After a couple of doses of morphine, we got a chance to look at the leg properly. The ulceration was extensive across most of her calf, and right down to bone and tendons – not a pretty sight for the faint-hearted. It was clear the priority was pain control, but equally we could see that the only possible treatment was an amputation – but we doubted she was strong enough to survive that. She was sufficiently lucid to tell me that an amputation was not acceptable to her, and all she wanted was to be out of pain. So, the treatment plan was clear. I explained to her that she was unlikely to survive this. It was a relief to see her relax and become more comfortable as we cared for her and settled her pain. She died less than two days later.

Ars Moriendi

In the Middle Ages a set of publications termed *Ars Moriendi* (the art of dying) became popular and widely read across Europe. It is thought that a Dominican monk wrote the first long version in around 1415, and many other versions followed. The text taught that dying was not to be feared, because of the promise of a better life after death. It described the five temptations of a dying man and how to avoid them: greed and material possessions; doubt and lack of faith; despair; impatience; and pride. At that time many people were illiterate, and so *Ars Moriendi* was also produced in paired woodcuts which illustrated the temptations and the remedies – a picture book on how to live and die. By breaking down death and dying into manageable steps and tasks, it helped focus the energy of a dying person and provide a sense of control. At that time, Christians had a strong view of the journey of life being a pilgrimage towards God's forgiveness and salvation in heaven. This was later portrayed by John Bunyan in *Pilgrim's Progress*, written in 1677, describing the temptations and snares of false paths for the traveller named 'Christian' on the journey to the Celestial City. Christian had to learn about patience and endurance. Later chapters in *Ars Moriendi* also describe how to console a dying man, the correct behaviour at the deathbed, and the prayers to be said. In *Being Mortal*, and perhaps with reference to the traditions such as *Ars Moriendi*, Atul Gawande says:[136]

> *In the past few decades, medical science has rendered obsolete centuries of experience, tradition, and language about our mortality, and created a new difficulty for mankind: how to die.*

A good death

What makes a good death today? We probably recognise it when we see it. Joy, in the introduction to this book, certainly exemplified it. Through the COVID pandemic we were confronted with a rather horrific picture of death in intensive care units on our TV screens night after night. It seems unlikely this did anything to reduce our innate fear of death. Perhaps this was intentional, to frighten us into obeying the lockdown restrictions... But it may have stimulated conversations about what we ourselves feel would be a good death. As a starting point, many of us might say it would be to die at home surrounded by our loved ones, and free of pain. But it would be foolish to try to generalise for something which for each of us is so unique and personal a journey. The Greek for a good death is *euthanasia*, yet that word today has quite different connotations. Interestingly, the former Euthanasia Society renamed itself some years ago 'Dying With Dignity', trying to convince us that a good death might require an act of assisted suicide. The importance of dignity in death chimes well with many of us, *sharing precious moments with those we love most.*

For many if not most, to die at peace will require acceptance – reflecting the steps in *Ars Moriendi*. Geriatricians know that half of their patients are probably in the last year of life. In assessing a new patient, I

---

[136] Gawande, Atul (2014); *Being Mortal;* p158 Profile Books.

would frequently say to myself, "What if this turned out to be her last month of life?" checking that I would have no regrets about our decisions if this were the case. Had I been honest enough in explaining the chances of recovery? Philip Gould in his book *When I Die – Lessons from the Death Zone*[137], wrote:

> *The doctors who matter, the doctors you trust, always confront this reality. They tell you sooner rather than later you are going to die... Only when you accept death can you free yourself from it, deal with it, move forward from it. Acceptance is the key. At that moment you gain freedom. You gain power. You gain courage.*

The encounter I described in chapter five with Muriel after her scan result illustrated this; she was able to see a positive way forward although I was unable to offer treatment.

Death trajectories

There were 760,000 deaths in the UK in 2020; a third were aged over eighty-five, and just over half were aged over seventy-five at the time of death. For those dying aged over eighty, the leading cause of death is now dementia in twenty percent, followed by chest infections in eleven percent, heart disease in ten percent and strokes in seven percent.[138] If all forms of cancer are combined, rather than treated as separate diseases, cancer deaths amount to around fifteen percent of deaths in the over eighty-fives. The official statistics rarely include 'old age' as the cause of death – nor do many obituaries. Doctors are permitted to write "Old Age" as the cause of death but prefer to write something more 'medical'. The trajectory of death is quite different for these different causes. Death from cancer may be predictable as health steadily declines over some months, while a death from a stroke or heart attack is quite sudden and unpredictable. Long term diseases are characterised by recurring acute, sometimes life-threatening episodes, followed by a recovery until the final episode that proves fatal. Death from an infection may occur over a matter of days. But for all these causes, where death occurs in the context

---

[137] Gould, Philip (2012); *When I Die – Lessons from the Death Zone;* Little, Brown book group; p.118

[138] Office for National Statistics (2016); 'Deaths registered in England and Wales (series DR)'; Office for National Statistics; ons.gov.uk

of advancing frailty, health has been deteriorating for a long time. This makes predicting how long someone with frailty has still to live, or when the last illness will happen, very difficult indeed.

Despite the growth of palliative care, hospices and the Macmillan service, only a quarter of all deaths occur at home and six percent in a hospice. For the over eighty-fives, the percentages are forty-three percent in hospital, thirty-eighty percent in care homes, eighteen percent at home and one percent in a hospice. The trends over the last twenty years have seen a gradual fall in the percentage of hospital deaths along with a gradual rise in the care home,[139] and the COVID pandemic saw a further reduction in hospital deaths.

Dying with frailty in a time of COVID

In 2020, the world was stopped in its tracks by COVID. The oldest and most frail in our communities were hit the hardest, bearing seventy-five percent or more of the deaths. A quarter of all the deaths were in care homes. Deaths in 2020 were fourteen percent higher for men over eighty-five, and ten percent higher for women over eighty-five, than a couple of years earlier. Many of the COVID deaths were in extreme old age and dementia, and therefore could be seen as a natural end. For some with frailty, lives may well have been cut short by the virus, perhaps even by years, but many were also ready for their life to end. Kate Clanchy[140] movingly described the deaths of her parents during the pandemic, both of whom had strong views about advance care plans:

> ...both my parents become statistics on the news. They are in so many ways typical COVID victims – exactly the median age with a number of co-morbidities – that I feel I should be able find them in those numbers, mourn them when the nation stands in silence and puts out flags for the fallen. It's hard, though. My parents weren't fighting that war. If COVID shortened their lives, it was not by much: the loneliness of lockdown hit them harder. They did not want to combat death: they were trying to let it in, to find a human way to go.

---

[139] https://www.gov.uk/government/publications/end-of-life-care-profiles-february-2018-update/statistical-commentary-end-of-life-care-profiles-february-2018-update

[140] 'Letting go: my battle to help my parents die a good death'; *The Guardian*

Those living with frailty had to bear the hardship of isolation, shielding and prolonged lockdown. This was particularly tough for those with dementia whose insight was reduced, and for whom contact with their family was such a critical lifeline and hold on reality. Many of those admitted to hospital would die without their family present, or only visiting in their last hours as they were slipping away. Some families were too scared to visit. Most older people living with frailty were identified as having no chance of surviving a gruelling spell on a ventilator in ITU, and so were looked after in dedicated wards equipped with oxygen and palliative care. And thankfully not all succumbed. For bereaved families, a further sadness was the greatly curtailed funeral and remembrance services so important for saying goodbye.

Through all of this, were we asking what older people wanted themselves? For many, life without family contact probably no longer seemed worth living. It is likely that many would have opted for continued family visits, even if this did mean a risk of catching the virus from them. But of course, for those living in care homes, allowing visitors risked spreading the virus more widely to other residents who might have chosen differently.

Death will always have a sadness, but it is not necessarily tragic. As I write, we have recently heard of the death of Captain Tom, who died at the age of a hundred, having raised millions of pounds for the NHS in his last year of life. He wrote shortly before his death from COVID, "There is something almost reassuring about accepting the decline that I cannot prevent. A kind of calmness overcomes you when you realise that the end might come at any time. Death becomes somehow easier to think about, and not something to be afraid of."[141]

Dying with frailty in hospital

For almost half of the over eighty-fives, many still living at home, their last days are spent in hospital following an emergency admission. For some, decisions had been made that when facing a probable final illness, their preference was to be in hospital. This might be because their partner could not face seeing the last days and hours close at hand. We often felt sad about this in the hospital, wondering if, with palliative care support including having someone staying in the house with them, a

---

[141] *The Times;* February 23rd, 2021

peaceful death at home would have been perfectly feasible. For many others, there had been no agreed plan and hospital was the default in a crisis.

Listening to the patient letting go

Sometimes it is the patient who indicates quite clearly they have had enough and are letting go.

June was eighty-four years old when I met her for the second time. She had chronic obstructive pulmonary disease – COPD – which we used to call chronic bronchitis. She came into hospital from time to time with her lung disease. She was breathless much of the time, had oxygen at home and was confined to the house. I was talking to her on the ward after she had recovered from the latest severe attack, and we were reviewing the support she had at home. Then, somewhat out of the blue, she said, "Couldn't you just end my life for me?" Well, of course, no I couldn't, but we chatted about how she felt. She explained that she had not really wanted to be treated this time but didn't know how to say this. I spoke with her family, who said she had felt like ending her life for quite some time now and would speak about this at home. I realised this was a settled view of hers and her family, and we agreed to complete an advance care plan which said she would not have life-saving antibiotics again. It was only a week later, and while she was still on the ward waiting for her homecare to restart, that a further hospital-acquired infection started. She remained adamant about the antibiotics, and she died two days later, with treatment to relieve her breathlessness.

We had been slow to listen to June until she was the one courageous enough to speak. Much depends on communication and trust; surely the best way is when doctor and patient both trust and understand each other sufficiently for difficult conversations to happen.

Tom sadly illustrates a more common scenario.

Tom was eighty-two years old and was admitted to hospital because of coughing and breathlessness. He had suffered a severe bout of vomiting the day before. His chest X-ray revealed a pneumonia. This was his third admission this year with something similar. This time he became confused and was hardly eating. His kidney function deteriorated, and over the next few weeks he needed prolonged intravenous fluids, which was difficult with his restless disturbed behaviour. He then developed diarrhoea which was identified as *Clostridium difficile* – a notorious bug which can complicate a course of high dose antibiotics. Now all dignity was lost. After four exhausting weeks, he finally died in hospital, with his family denied visiting because of the diarrhoea bug.

There is a moment when doctors let go of the hope of cure. All deaths in hospital are reviewed by what is called a 'mortality and morbidity review' – these meetings also review serious adverse events which did not end in death. In our elderly care department, we always found the process beneficial, and one of the most frequent conclusions was that we could have seen death coming sooner. The implication was that if we had recognised this, then our management would have been a little different, suffering might have been less, and the family would have had more time to say goodbye.

Just exhausted with hospital care

Some of those living with frailty have had enough of hospital care and being 'messed about' and want to be left alone. This may not be a settled view but reflects how hard it is to endure a long period of treatment in hospital.

Angela was aged seventy-eight years, but was old for her years because of her severe disfiguring rheumatoid arthritis. She had battled on and had her home well set up for her disability. She had been on my ward for three weeks with a fluctuating fever, and we could not identify the source of her infection. She had been given lots of intravenous antibiotics and had very sore arms from numerous drips. The blood tests were not getting any better. Then I decided to repeat the scan of her liver, and this time it showed two abscesses not spotted two weeks earlier. Finally, we had something which could give her a cure, as the abscesses could be drained and the fluid cultured. I gave her the news, and she said no, she would not agree to the operation to drain the abscesses. This was a Friday, and she also refused further antibiotics. I came back in on Monday half expecting to hear she might have died, but she was there. She said she had changed her mind and would agree to the drainage. All proceeded smoothly, and she recovered. When I met her two months later, she said, "I know, I was silly, I'm sorry."

Some deaths seem to follow a giving up and letting go – turning your face to the wall, we might say. This seems more common in extreme old age and might sometimes cause the doctor difficulty in describing the cause of death. How often have partners followed each other into the grave, even where no serious illness was known – they just didn't want to go on any longer. I recall talking to a seventy-nine-year-old lady on the ward who had suffered quite a severe stroke four weeks earlier and had not recovered any walking. She still needed hoisting into her chair and onto the toilet. Her husband had died three months earlier. Our team discussed the options with her, and we concluded that she would need to live in a nursing home for the care she required. She reluctantly agreed with a heavy heart. But from that day on she turned her face to the wall and stopped eating. Her strength left her, and she died three weeks later.

Waiting

Some are left just waiting for a final illness. Those living with severe frailty are likely to have at least one emergency admission each year, but not necessarily with a life-threatening illness. Kathryn Mannix, in her beautiful and illuminating book *With the End in Mind*, described a case of a ninety-six-year-old lady who was being treated successfully for abdominal pain due to severe constipation.[142] The palliative care consultant explored her thoughts for the future:

> *'Do you wish to be dead?' I ask her, and she pauses to think before telling me that she does not wish deliberately to end her life but regrets that she has lived past being useful and mobile. I nod and reflect that she is naming a key difficulty of older age.*

I often met this tiredness of life, rather different from depression. It might be linked with a sense of satisfaction, having achieved what they wanted in life, with nothing to look forward to. "I've had my life," was a comment I heard, sometimes set beside, "Don't you worry about me."

---

[142] Mannix, Kathryn (2017); *With the End in Mind: Dying, Death and Wisdom in an Age of Denial;* HarperCollins; p.312

Where there is no imminent threat to life, I, like Kathryn Mannix, can only listen and offer empathy.

One disease often linked with years of 'existence' and waiting is dementia, particularly Alzheimer's disease. Even in severe disease where there is complete loss of speech and mobility, survival for several years can be expected if no other disease supervenes. This creates a prolonged spell of waiting which is extremely hard for the family to bear or make sense of.

Can letting go become euthanasia?

Sometimes it is the family who come and ask that we "let Dad go". Typically, the family will have gathered and asked for a meeting with the doctor. We would squash into the ward day room, and I would be joined by a senior nurse and a junior doctor, as we all introduced ourselves. Then the spokesperson for the family would say something like, "Look doc, we know Dad and we can see he's had enough. He can't face any more needles and drips. Can't you just let him go now? But don't let him suffer any more – he's suffered enough in these last weeks." And nine times out of ten, we would all agree about stopping active treatment such as antibiotics. But I wonder if we have a nagging worry that this is giving licence to some sort of euthanasia? That in stopping the antibiotics and drips, and in ensuring 'Dad does not suffer any more', we are asking the doctor to tread a path that is hastening death? Perhaps as a Christian we feel uneasy about this?

Let's explore briefly what euthanasia is:

- *Voluntary euthanasia* is where, following a request from the patient, a doctor administers a drug which will end the person's life under his supervision. The specific and sole intent of the drugs or injection is to bring about the end of life.
- *Involuntary euthanasia* is where the patient is unable to make that request because they are now unconscious or too confused to do so. The patient may have made a written request previously, or the family are acting on behalf of the patient. Again, the doctor administers an injection with the sole intention of ending the person's life to end their suffering.
- *Physician assisted suicide* is where the doctor has prescribed some drugs which the patient will take themselves usually at a time and place of their choosing.

All of these are illegal in the UK, but each is legal in some countries today. The scenario we have just described is neither euthanasia nor physician-assisted suicide.

You may be surprised at the strength of support for euthanasia in surveys which include Christians. A British Social Attitudes survey found, in response to the question, "About a person with a painful incurable disease, do you think that doctors should be allowed, by law to end the patient's life, if the patient requests it?" those *against* were only nine percent of those declaring no religion, fourteen percent of Anglicans and twenty-nine percent of Catholics. Those figures have gradually dropped from 1983 to 2012.[143] The latest survey in 2016 showed that overall, eighty-nine percent without religion and sixty-seven percent with religion supported euthanasia for those with a terminal illness.[144] Older people themselves have lower rates of acceptance, and in the Netherlands few people over eighty have requested euthanasia. The British Medical Association's latest survey of doctors in 2020 regarding physician-assisted suicide[145] found overall that forty percent of doctors would like to see this permitted by law; conversely, forty-five percent of all doctors were *not* willing to assist themselves, and this increased to fifty-six percent of geriatricians and seventy-six percent of palliative care consultants.

Patients cannot insist on being given a drug to end their life through an advance care plan, nor through a lasting power of attorney. At the start of this chapter, I described Doreen who came to us in terrible pain. We gave her strong drugs to relieve pain and her terrible suffering. The intention of those drugs was solely to relieve the pain. There can be worries of a so-called double-effect – that those drugs may at the same time hasten death. This would not be euthanasia, because the drugs were not given with the sole purpose of ending a life. It is true that if the drugs were given in far too high a dosage, there is a greater risk of them hastening death – so the doctor is legally accountable for using appropriate knowledge and skill, as with any medicine. The relief of pain

---

[143] British Religion in Numbers (2014); 'Religion and attitudes towards euthanasia in Britain: Evidence from opinion polls and social surveys'; brin.ac.uk

[144] British Social Attitudes Survey 34 (2016); bsa34_moral_issues_final.pdf; natcen.ac.uk

[145] BMA survey on assisted dying (2020); 'Kantar Public Division Physician-assisted dying survey'; bma.org.uk

or breathlessness or anxiety allows the person to relax finally and be at peace, which then enables them to let go. It is in that spirit that we can pray – doctors, nurses, family – on behalf of our loved one, as active treatment is stopped, "Lord, let thy servant depart in peace," and reassure them they can let go into the arms of God.

"You're just letting him starve to death"

Some people are ready to let go of their hold on life; other families are more concerned that the medical staff have given up on their relative. They may be concerned whether Mum or Dad is eating and drinking enough.

Elizabeth was a retired English teacher who had enjoyed good health for most of her life. She had developed Alzheimer's seven years ago, and it rapidly deteriorated after her husband died. Seven years on and the picture was rather different – she had moved into a care home after two years, and now her family said she barely recognised them. Yet she seemed contented and happy, and the staff looked after her well. In the last year she had lost interest in her food, and the staff had to cajole her to eat. I met her when she came to hospital with concern about losing weight and perhaps being dehydrated. She was seen by the speech therapist who noted that her swallowing was unsafe, and food would often go the wrong way, even though choking had not really been noticed by the nurses. Her CT brain scan showed up several small strokes, which we decided was the cause for her faulty swallow reflex. We explained the situation to her family – her son and daughter – that she was eating too little to survive, and the only treatment option would be to place a feeding tube known as a PEG – percutaneous endoscopic gastrostomy. Her daughter felt her mother would not want her life prolonged any further, but her son was terribly upset at the thought of "Mum starving to death". After two emotionally draining meetings, we decided not to place a feeding tube, although her son remained unhappy with the decision. She died in a local hospital a few weeks later – and we waited to see if a complaint letter arrived from the son. Thankfully, it never materialised.

I have observed so often this loss of interest in food, and indeed refusal to eat, in those with advancing dementia. Loss of appetite is a normal part of the dying process, and hunger fades as quickly as after a week of not eating. It is as if some signal in their body is telling them to let go. Losing weight in dementia is a strong predictor of the last months of life. Research has found that inserting feeding tubes in situations like Elizabeth's hardly prolongs life at all. This is partly because the risk of pneumonia from aspirating liquids in the stomach continues just the same with or without the feeding tube. But it may also be because life is coming to a natural end.

In situations like Elizabeth's, I have seen medical staff place a 'nil by mouth' sign above the bed to ensure no food goes the wrong way and starts a pneumonia. But this apparent concern can be cruel, and was certainly not understood by Elizabeth. Paul Hobbs, a Christian artist, has a picture entitled 'Nil by Mouth'[146] (you can see the picture online) with this explanation:

> *An old man, seemingly stripped of his worth by illness and frailty, wears a halo that suggests his eternal value in the eyes of God. The man's isolation from his fellow man can remind us that the difference between happiness and misery in old age is not so much to do with the state of one's health, as the state of one's relationships with others and whether you are loved.*

Whether waiting is long or short, we need to be reminded that God continues to love the person perhaps trapped inside their failing body or mind.

Thirst at the end of life

When it seems that survival is unlikely, and little is being swallowed, there can be discussion about the value of giving fluids artificially by a dripped infusion. Attending relatives would love to tell me on a ward round how their Mum woke for a moment while they lovingly cajoled her to take a little to drink. But are the dying distressed by thirst?

Perhaps as Christians we can identify with Christ's cry on the cross, "I thirst,"[147] and hope that suffering may be relieved a little by a drink… Palliative nurses are convinced that this thirst derives from the dry sensation in the mouth more than actual dehydration, and so keeping the mouth moist is of greatest value. If drinking is difficult, sips or fluid on a sponge can be helpful.

---

[146] Paul Hobbs; 'Nil by Mouth'; arthobbs.com
[147] John 19:28 (NIV)

Is denying artificial fluids hastening the death – would fluids by a drip prolong life a little? The General Medical Council provides ethical guidance to doctors on these matters.[148] They advise that doctors should weigh up the likely benefits and burdens of providing artificial nutrition and fluids. The benefit might be in treating a reversible problem such as a high blood sugar causing symptoms, while the burden would be the need for a needle, blood tests and the possible prolongation of the dying process. Continuing artificial fluids in the absence of nutrition will often lead to marked body swelling with fluid. This swelling can be extreme, which can be distressing as well as damaging the skin. In the last days of life, the burdens usually exceed any possible benefit. But where the death may still be some weeks away, then support may be helpful.

Is there a case for euthanasia in frailty?

In the previous chapter, we saw that by choosing a lasting power of attorney or writing an advance care plan, we can have a degree of control over illnesses at the end of life, if we have been brave enough to talk things through. We can reasonably trust that our doctors at home and in the hospital will treat us wisely and will not use treatments which are more burdensome than beneficial. It is often hard to predict with certainty how an acute illness will end – there have been plenty of times I have been surprised to see the patient very much alive the next day. But by not intervening aggressively, I have allowed events to take their natural course one way or another.

The stronger case for euthanasia is where no acute illness happens and yet there is much suffering and a deeply felt desire for life to be over. For the Christian, we try to seek comfort from feeling that our time has just not yet come to be 'called home'. Many will argue that Jesus demonstrated situation ethics – what is the most loving thing I can do in this situation, regardless of the rules? Paul Badham concluded his examination of whether there is a Christian case for euthanasia with the following:[149]

---

[148] GMC (2010); 'Treatment and care towards the end of life'; treatment-and-care-towards-the-end-of-life---english-1015_pdf-48902105.pdf; gmc-uk.org

[149] Badham, Paul (2009); *Is There a Christian Case for Assisted Dying?*; SPCK; p.121

When people's sufferings are so great that they make repeated requests to die, it sems a denial of that loving compassion, which is supposed to be the hallmark of Christianity, to refuse to allow their requests to be granted. If we truly love our neighbour as ourselves how can we deny them the death we would wish for ourselves in such a condition? We might also note that St Paul believed that 'love does not insist on its own way'. This suggests that love might require us to assist a person to die if that were their wish even if it were not ours.

I personally am not convinced. My concern, as with many, is that any legalisation of physician-assisted suicide would be the slippery slope that would encourage those who consider themselves to be a burden to their family making a request to end their life. You must decide yourself whether wise use of healthcare within the current laws, and as I have described throughout this book, can adequately reduce the perceived need for euthanasia for those living with severe frailty or dementia.

Dying with frailty and faith

Many patients I looked after assured me that their death would come as a relief, though many others were too ill or confused to have this degree of insight into their approaching death. We hope for a long life well lived and a legacy we are proud of. Life in the twenty-first century has made this possible for many – with one third of us living beyond eighty-five. We hope we have reached a place of peace with ourselves and our loved ones. We hope we have reached acceptance of our situation, and that healthcare has been a help and not an excessive burden through our last illnesses. We hope for a period of time, which may be quite brief, when we can see death coming and can make our goodbyes. If you wish to read more, I can strongly recommend Ann Clifford's book *Time To Live* as she describes "the beginner's guide to saying goodbye"[150].

Fear of dying is surely natural and probably inescapable, but we have explored through this book how choosing wisely the healthcare we receive can ensure we get the best out of our amazing national health service. I hope also that I have reduced the fear of being kept alive by overzealous medicine.

---

[150] Clifford, Ann (2017); *Time to Live: The Beginner's Guide to Saying Goodbye;* Instant Apostle

Christian faith can make an enormous difference to the fear in death: God does not want us to live in fear but in the certain hope for the future, the journey past death. In the introduction to this book, we met Joy. In the address at her commemoration, it was said of her, "I have fought the good fight; I have finished the race; I have kept the faith."[151] Most of us today will die at a good old age, and most of us will experience a time of frailty. I pray this book may have given you new insights into this contemporary dilemma of how to use healthcare wisely.

For you to consider

- Are you brave enough to talk honestly with those dearest to you about the healthcare you would like, or the healthcare you would like to refuse, towards the end of your life?
- Do you think there is a danger that doctors or close family might wish to continue medical treatments beyond any real value? Do you feel empowered to influence this?
- Are you feeling guilty about wishing that the life of someone you love was over? Try talking through these things with your GP.

---

[151] 2 Timothy 4:7 (NSRV)

Acknowledgements

I want to thank all those whose support have made this book possible.

First to all the staff in OPAL – our Older Persons Assessment and Liaison team at Gloucestershire Royal Hospital, and also to all the community matrons. We have journeyed together to develop a frailty service we can be proud of. Special thanks to my colleague Dr Sangeeta Kulkarni, and to Teresa (Senior Nurse) and Jane (Community Matron) for helping me recall some of the case histories.

Special thanks to Kate who gave me permission to talk about her mother in my introduction, and to Allan for sharing his own experience.

My thanks to Richard, Imogen and Jennie who were kind enough to read some early manuscripts and provide gentle advice.

My thanks to Benjamin Harris for his wonderful yet simple drawings which I feel have lightened the tone at the start of each chapter.

My thanks to Luke and the team at Onwards and Upwards who have shown such kindness and understanding to a novice author.

And of course greatest thanks are to my wife who has spent hours reading and re-reading early drafts, patiently explaining to me sentences which would be unintelligible to a non-medical reader and cheering me on at every stage.

Related Books from the Publisher

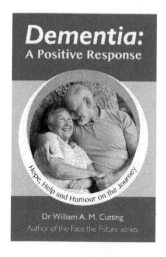

Dementia: A Positive Response
Dr William A. M. Cutting
ISBN: 978-1-78815-675-2

Those with dementia need and deserve much personal loving care! This book contains practical advice about how best to provide good and appropriate support. Whether you are someone with dementia, a personal carer, a family member or someone with a concern about the condition, you will find reasons for hope and positive encouragement. In simple language it sets out the current understanding about the condition and practical ways to help those living with the disease.

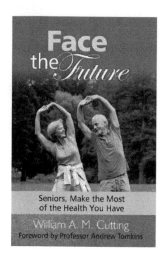

Face the Future: Seniors, Make the Most of the Health You Have
Dr William A. M. Cutting
ISBN: 978-1-910197-63-9

As well as providing helpful, easy-to-understand medical advice and practical suggestions, the book teaches how to make the best use of the existing health services. There are steps that Seniors can take to minimize future risks, including sensible eating, reasonable exercise, arranging a safe living environment, and a careful use of the right medication. With appropriate lifestyle changes, Seniors can enjoy good health and fitness.

Books available from all good bookshops
and from the publisher:

www.onwardsandupwards.org/**shop**